Looking Up

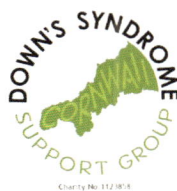

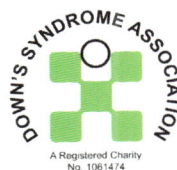

From Cornwall Down's Syndrome Support Group and the Down's Syndrome Association

ISBN: 978-0-9569367-3-8

Published by Coherent Visions, BCM Visions, London WC1N 3XX

Introduction from the Cornwall Down's Syndrome Support Group

Congratulations on the birth of your baby.

As parents of babies born with Down's Syndrome we all remember those early days after birth and for some of us the great need to find information on the future for our children.

The Looking Up groups are part of the Cornwall Down's Syndrome Support Group and the members wanted to reach out to other parents of newborns with Down's Syndrome to share positive and uplifting photos of the amazing journey of everyday life with their children. You will be facing some challenges ahead but in this book we do not focus on the medical facts or statistics but rather the children themselves.

At the back of this book are images of the wonderful Trisomy 21 exhibition which looks beyond the condition to the personalities of the child and young person.

We hope you enjoy looking at this book.

Sandy Lawrence | Cornwall Down's Syndrome Support Group

Introduction from the Down's Syndrorome Association (DSA)

Looking Up is the result of a brilliant new collaboration between the Cornwall Down's Syndrome Support Groups and the Down's Syndrome Association. In the book, we have featured pictorial stories following the early years in the lives of some of the children with Down's Syndrome in Cornwall.

Sometimes it can be really difficult for families to envisage what their new baby with Down's Syndrome will be like, particularly if he or she is born with health problems. This book helps to explode some of the myths and shows the reader that given the right opportunities, children with Down's Syndrome develop alongside their peers.

Carol Boys | CEO The Down's Syndrome Association

Acknowledgement

At the back of this book we have included photographs from the Trisomy 21 Exhibition which features some of the children of the Cornwall Down's Syndrome Support Group and was created by Simon Burt Photography.

www.simonburtphotography.co.uk

Funding for this project was provided by the Bolingey Barbarians – a group of mature rugby players who raise money for children's charities in Cornwall.

www.bolingey-barbarians.co.uk

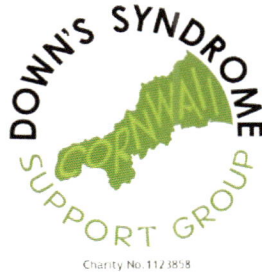

Cornwall Down's Syndrome Support Group

The Cornwall Down's Syndrome Support Group is a charity run by families affected by Down's Syndrome living in Cornwall.

We offer families a chance to meet, socialise and share information, friendship and support. Membership is free and we hold regular drop in sessions around the county where we can signpost our members to services that may be beneficial in an informal setting with entertainment for the children provided. During the year we organise many fun days out and trips away as well as our winter party. Our new parent support team warmly welcomes parents with a recent diagnosis.

Tel: 0751 1089267 | Email: info@cdssg.org.uk
www.cdssg.org.uk
© Down's Syndrome Association | Cornwall Down's Syndrome Support Group | Publication date: 2014

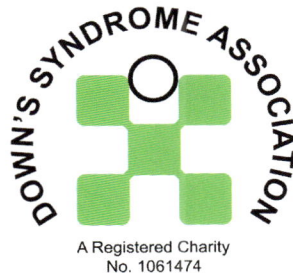

A Registered Charity
No. 1061474

The Down's Syndrome Association (DSA)

The Down's Syndrome Association provides information and support on all aspects of living with Down's syndrome. We also work to champion the rights of people with Down's syndrome, by campaigning for change and challenging discrimination. A wide range of Down's Syndrome Association publications can be downloaded free of charge from our website.

National Office
Langdon Down Centre, 2a Langdon Park, Teddington, Middlesex TW11 9PS.
Tel: 0333 1212 300 | Fax: 020 8614 5127 | E-mail: info@downs-syndrome.org.uk
www.downs-syndrome.org.uk

Wales
Suite 1, 206 Whitchurch Road, Heath, Cardiff CF14 3NB
Tel/Fax: 02920 522511

Northern Ireland
Unit 2, Marlborough House, 348 Lisburn Road, Belfast BT9 6GH
Tel: 02890 665260 Fax: 02890 667674

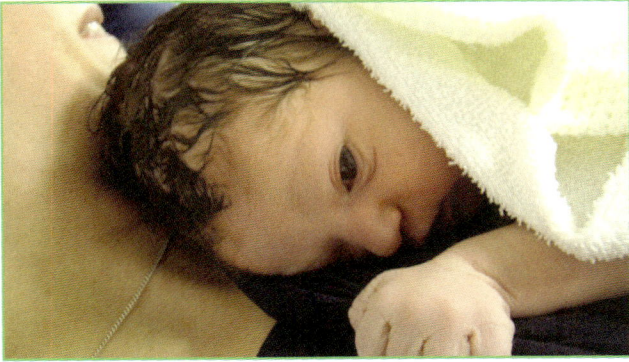

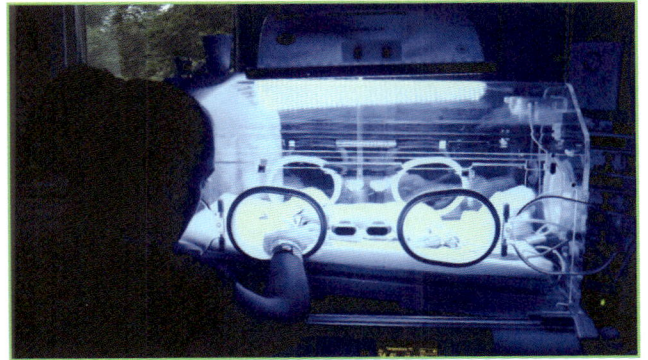

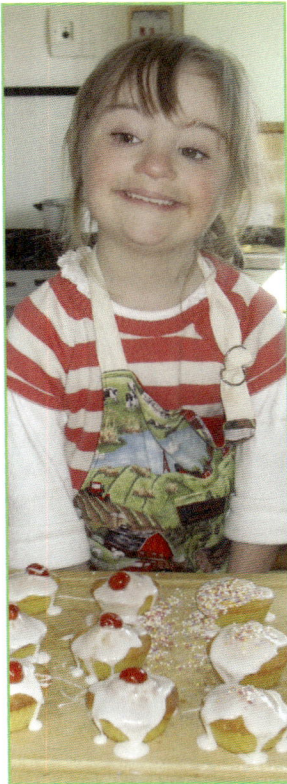

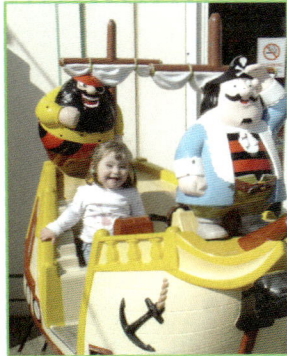

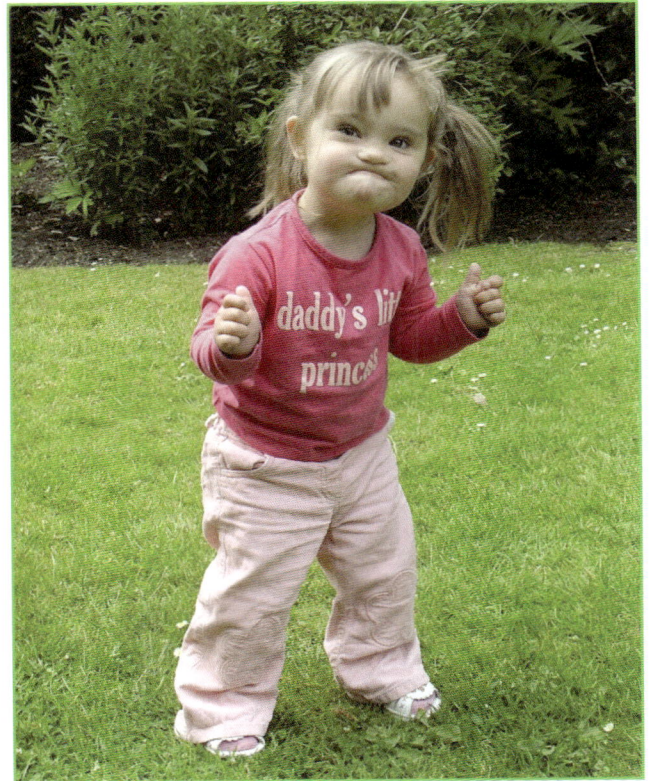

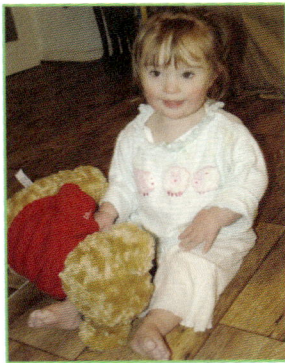

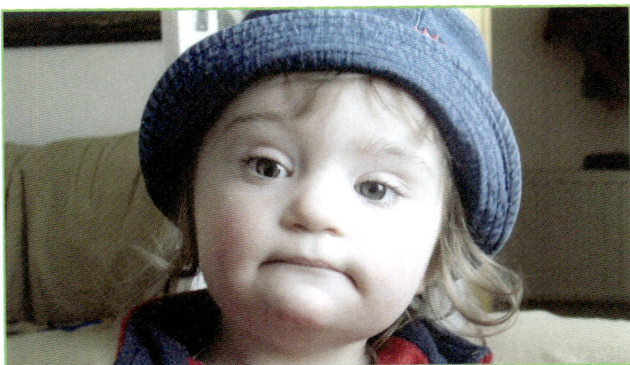

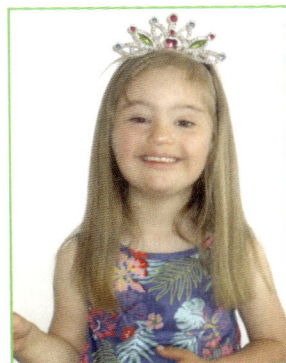

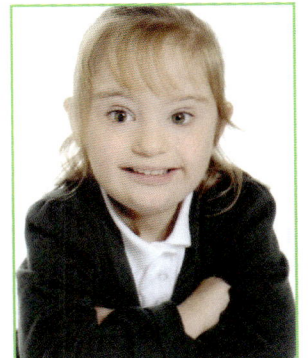

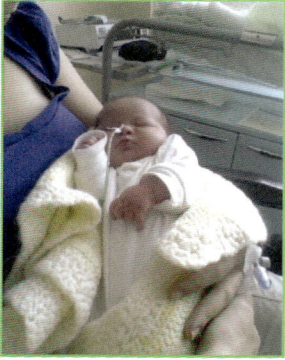
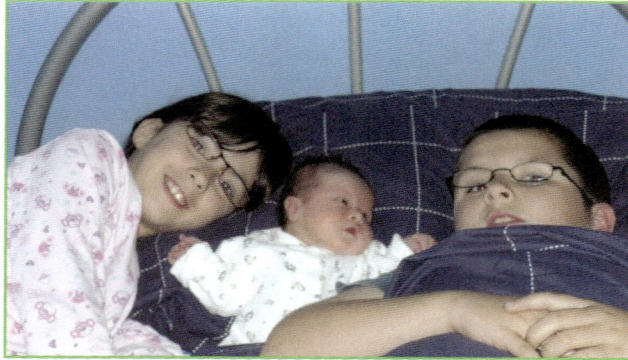
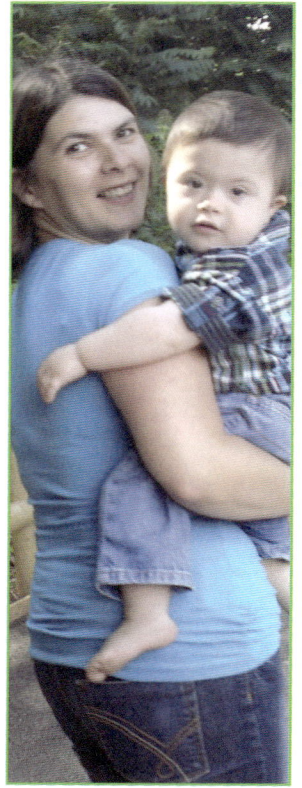
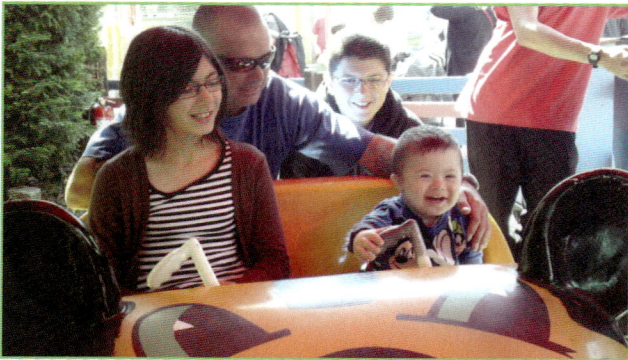
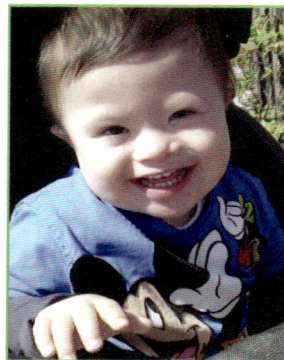
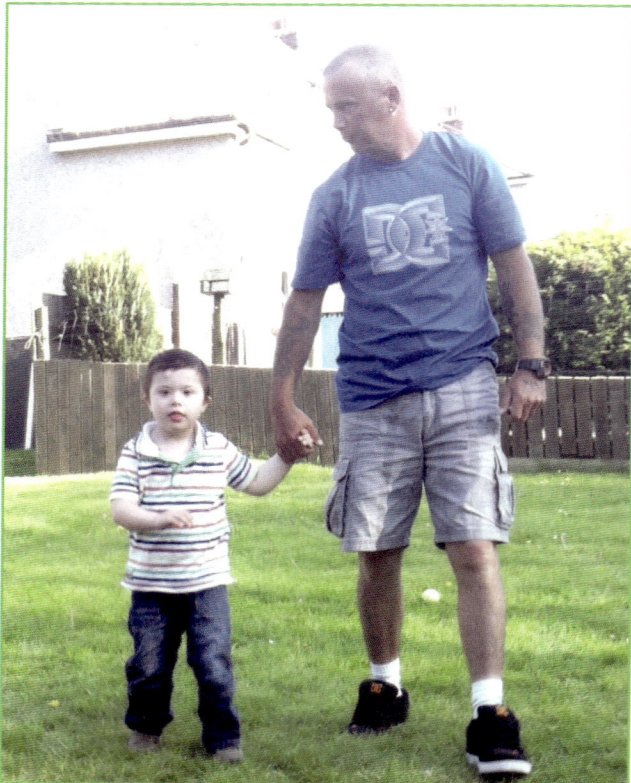
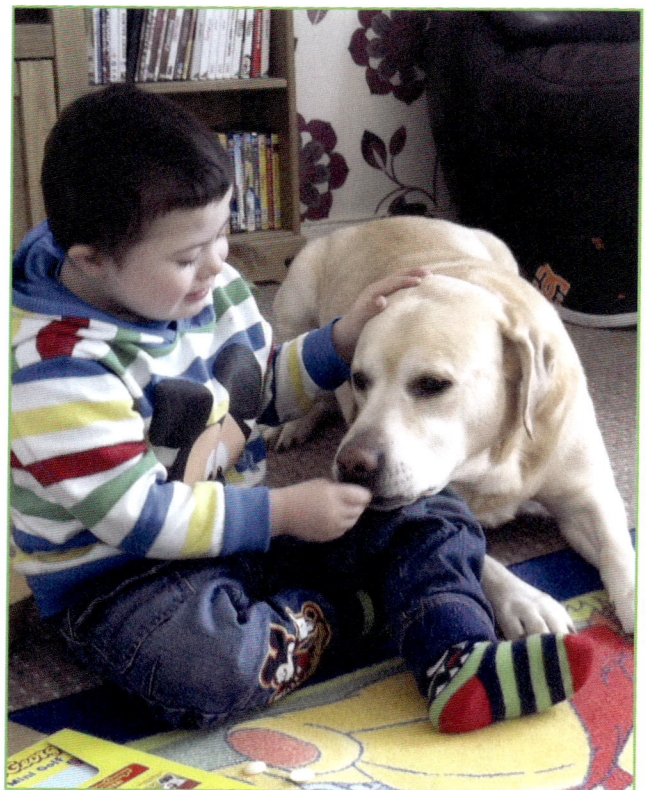

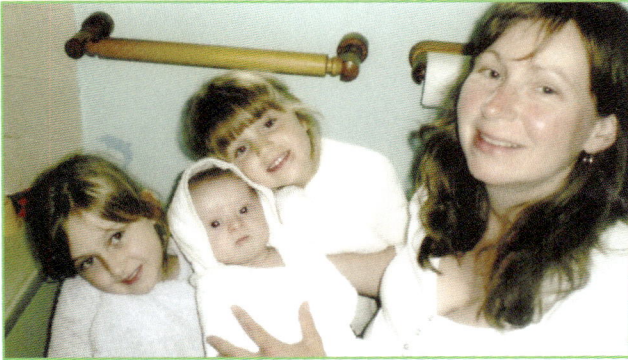
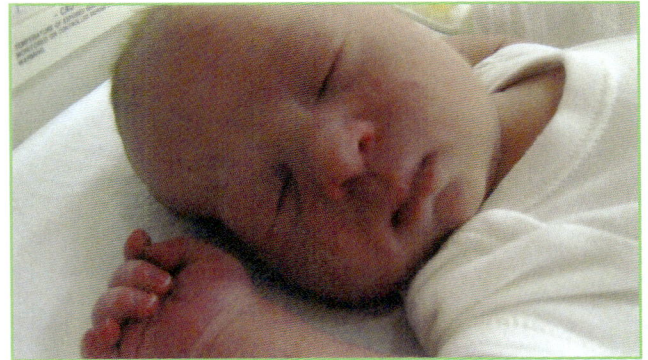
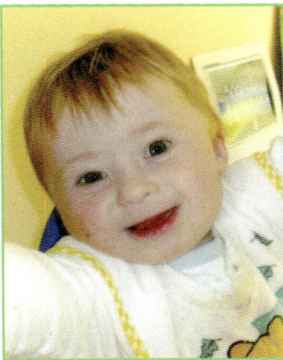
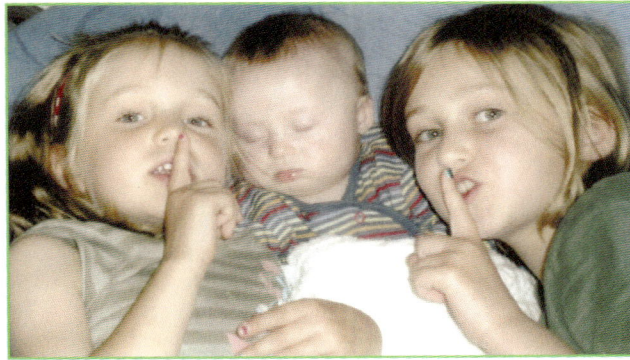
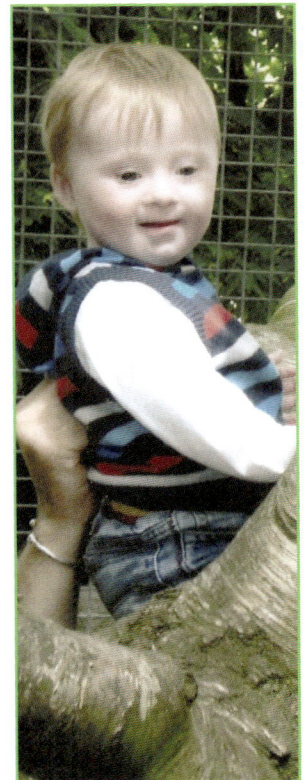
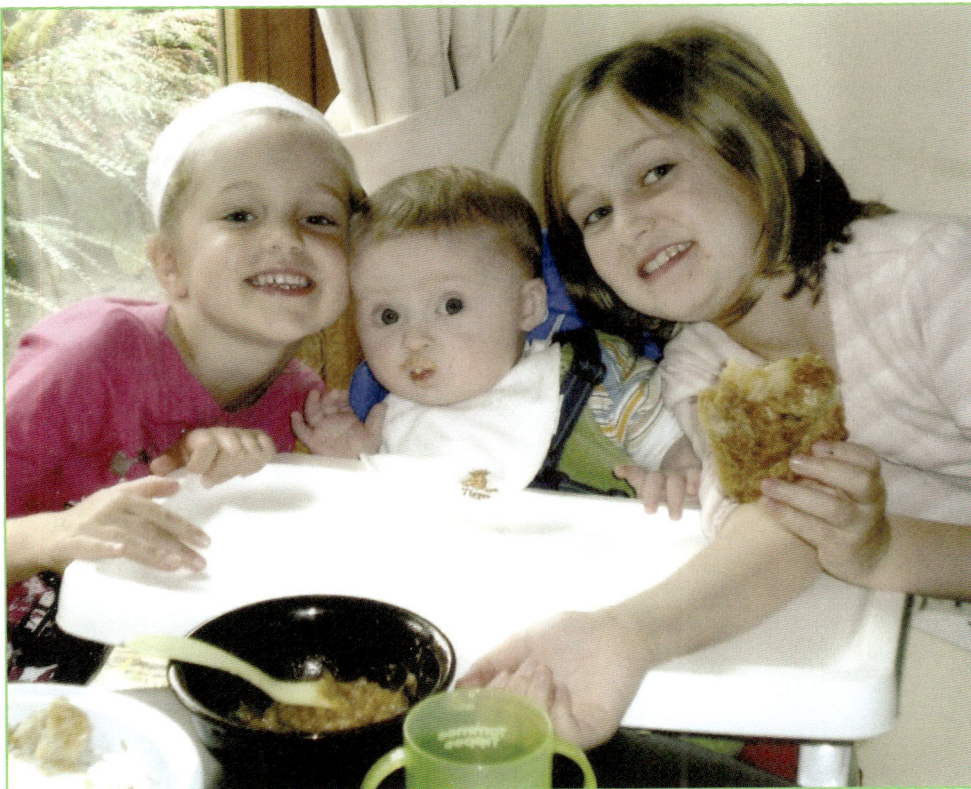
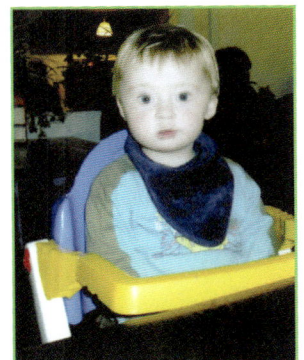

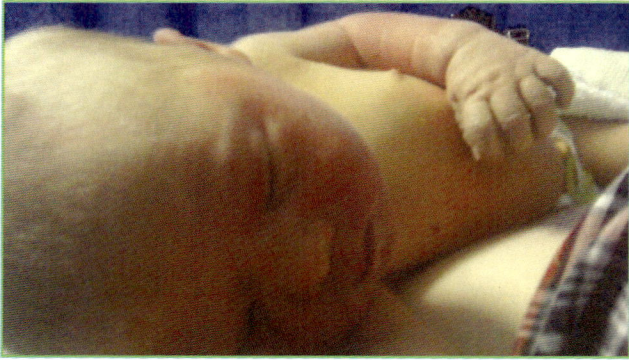

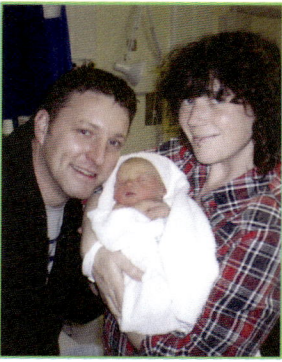

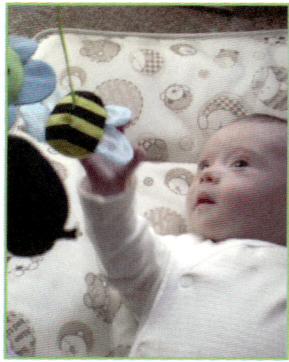

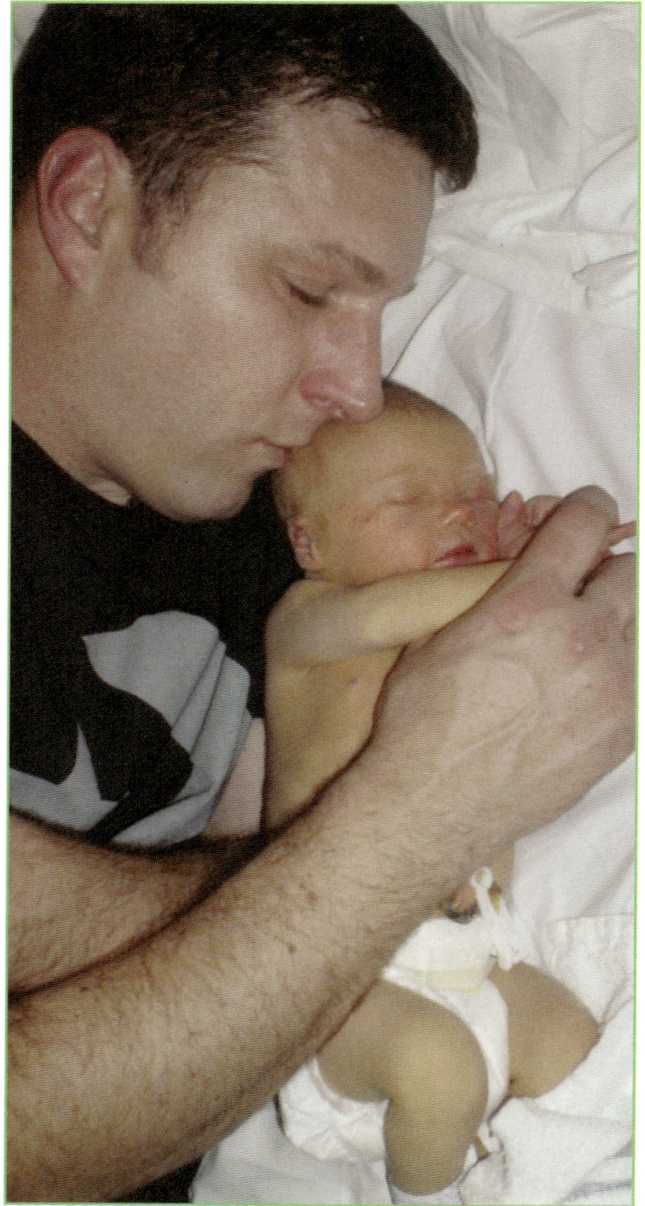

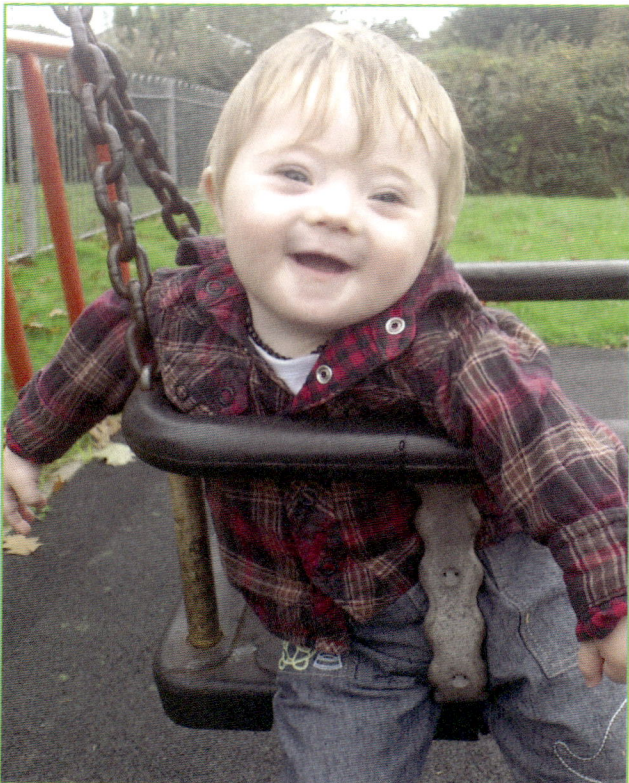

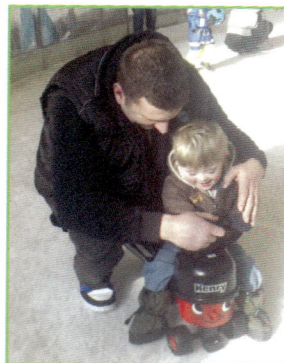

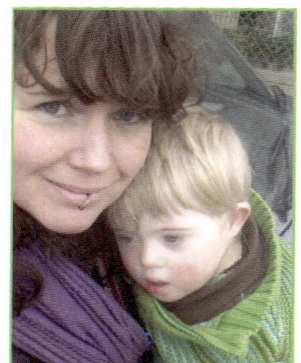

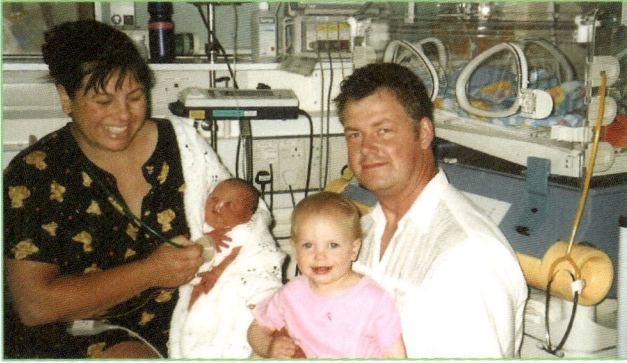
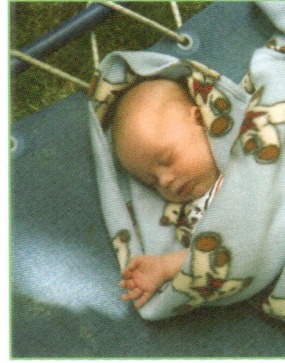
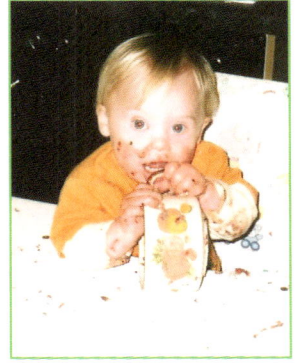
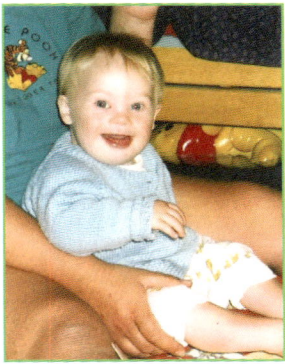
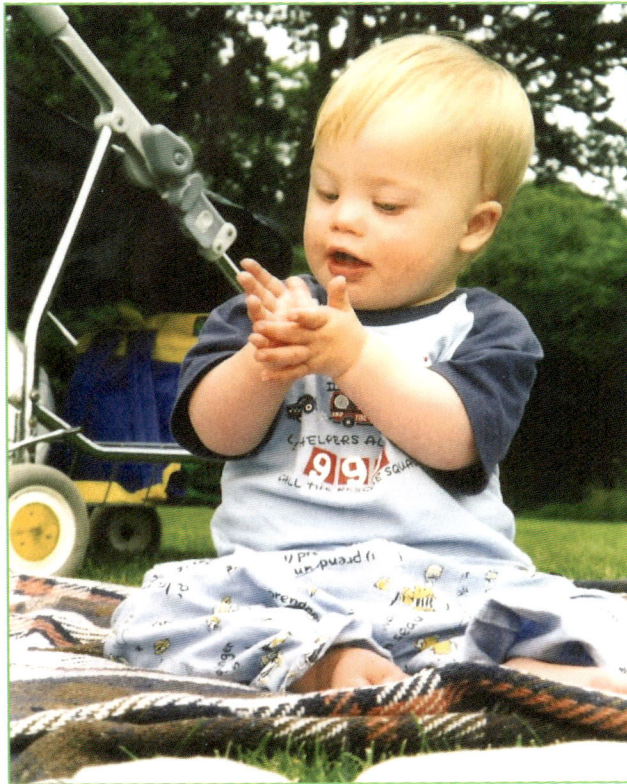
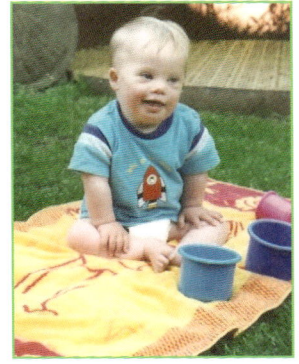
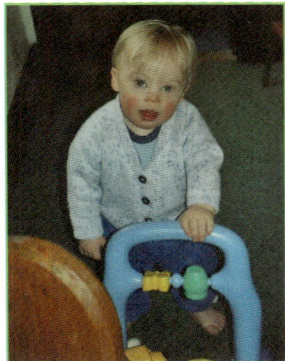
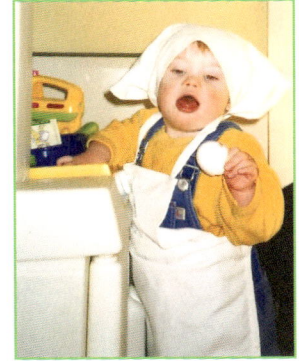
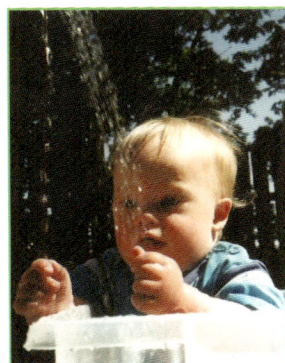
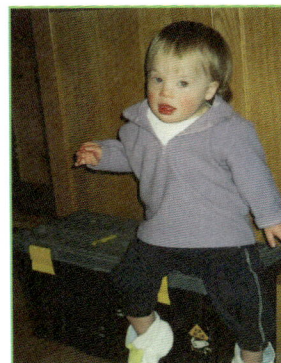
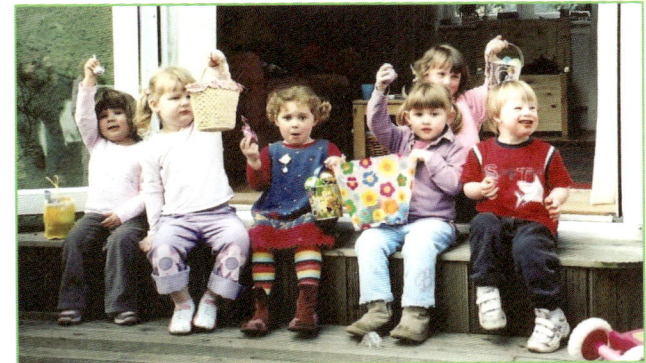

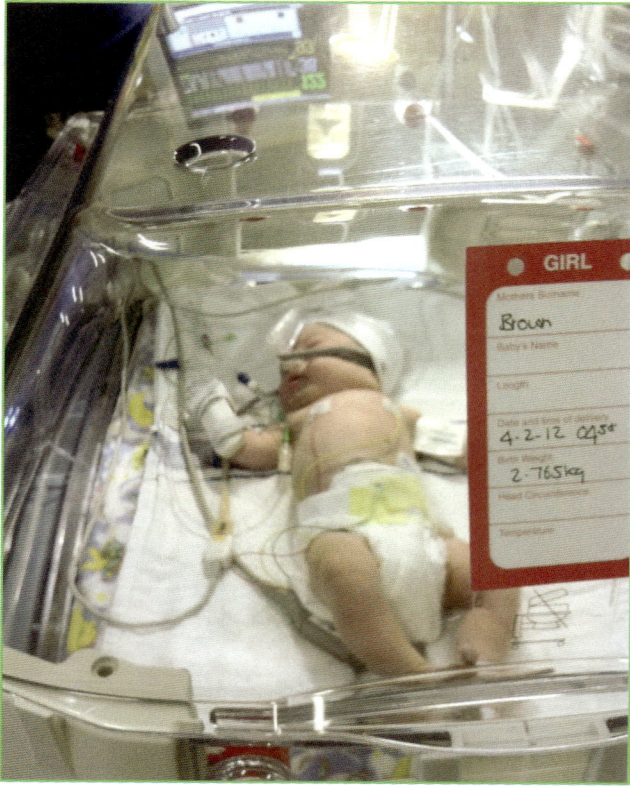

GIRL

Mothers Surname:
Brown

Baby's Name:

Length:

Date and time of delivery
4.2.12 04:35

Birth Weight
2.765kg

Head Circumference:

Temperature:

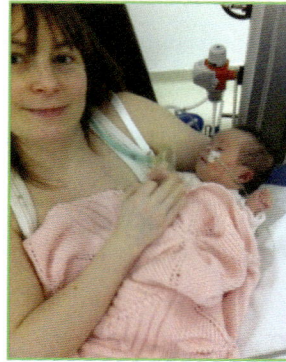

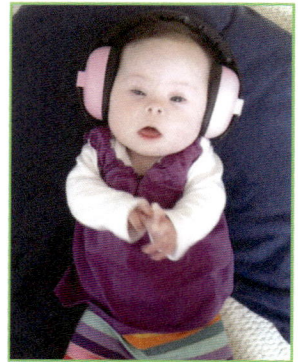

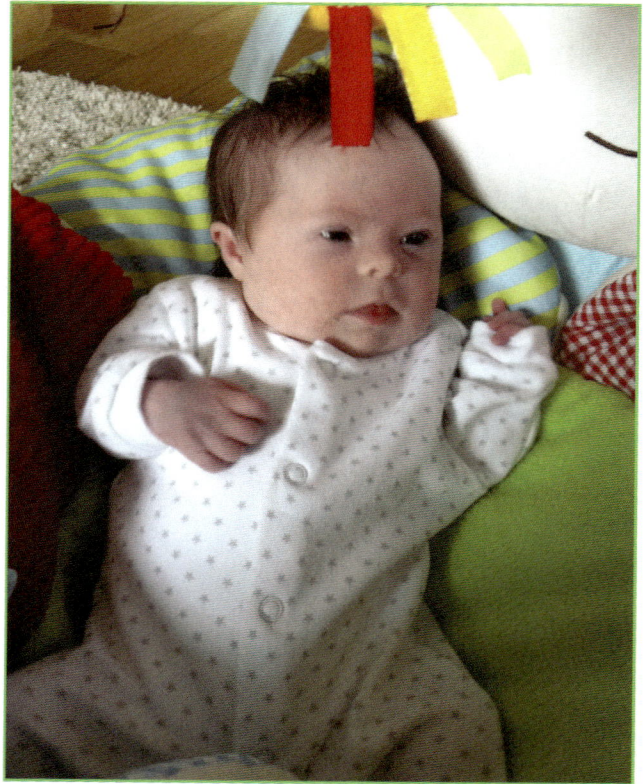

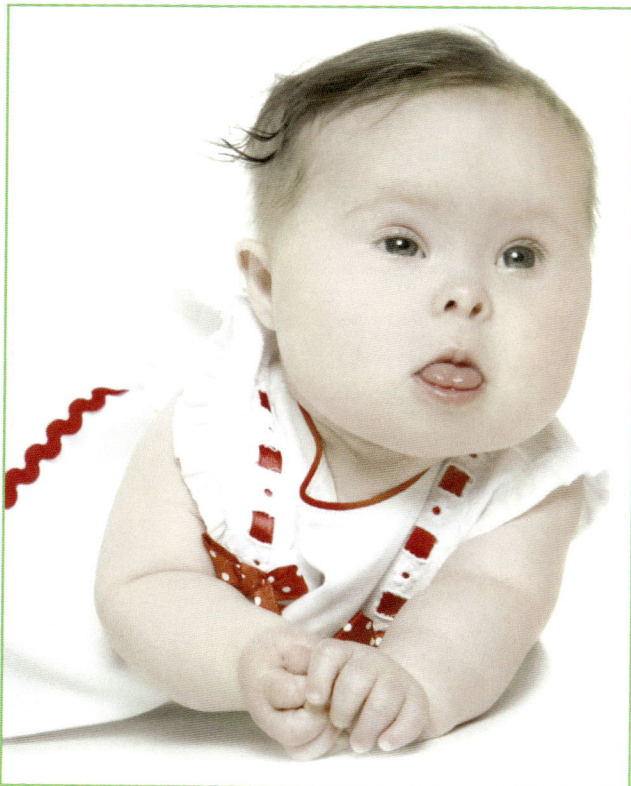

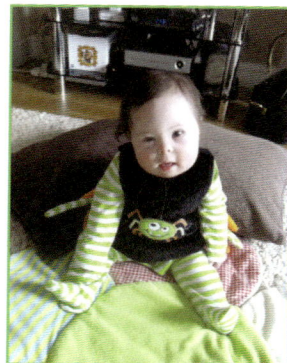

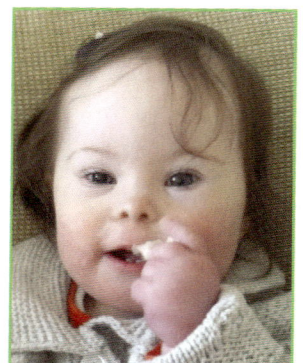

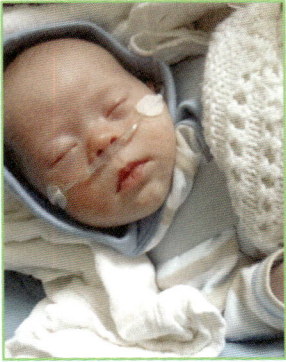
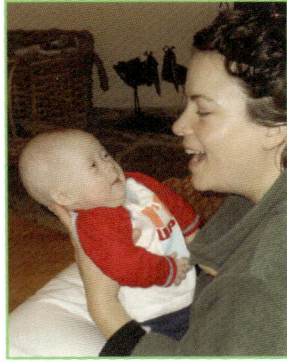
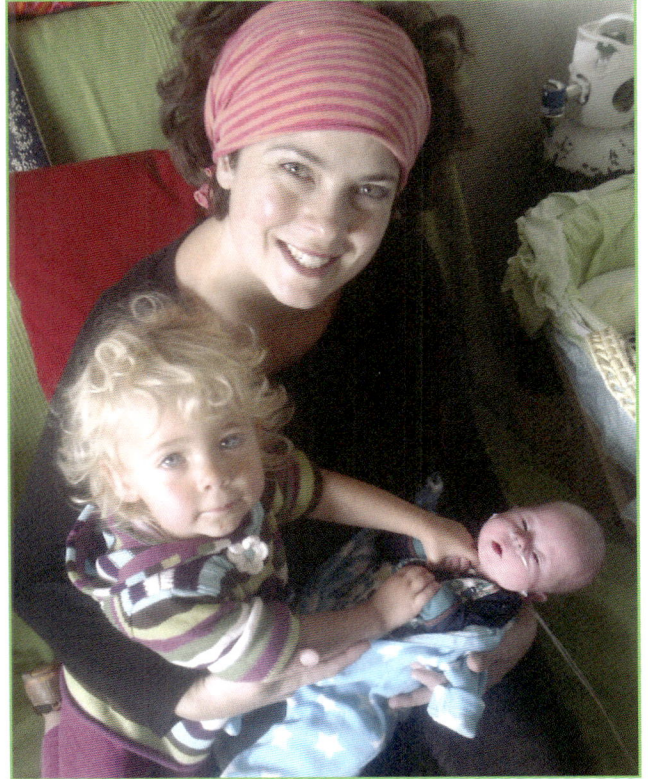
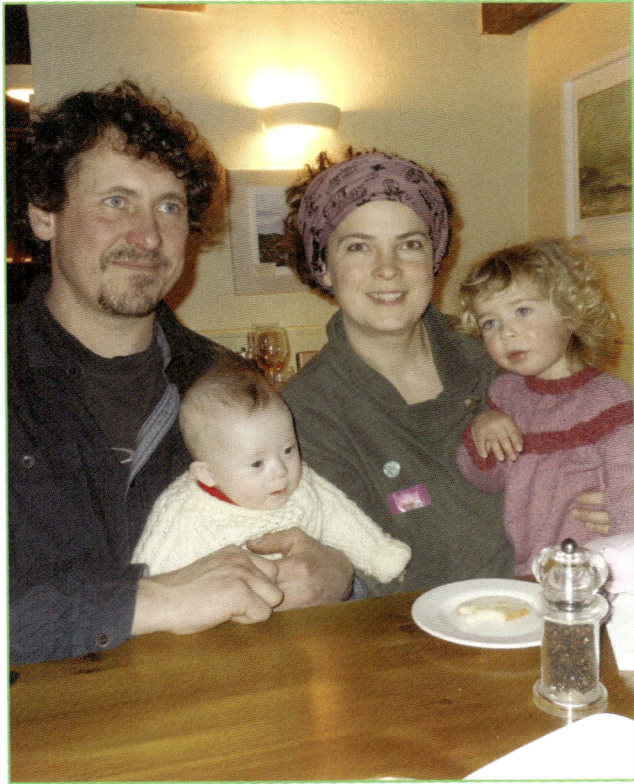
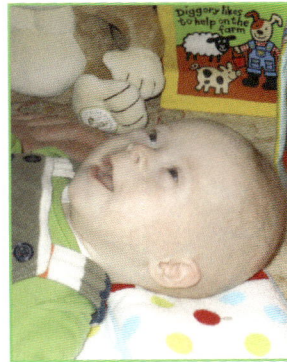
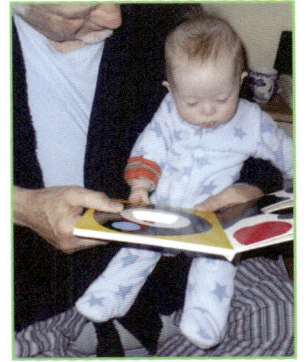
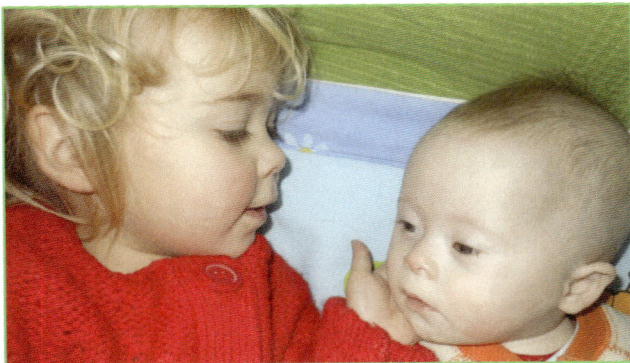
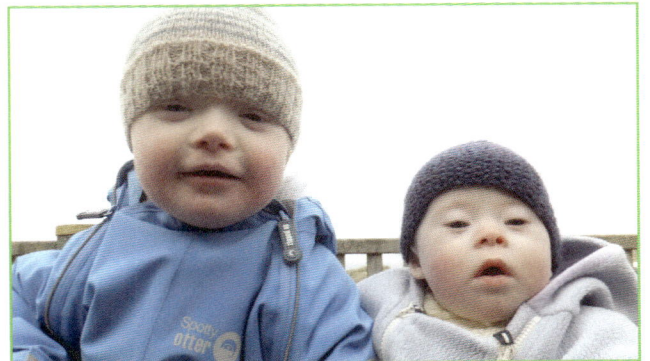

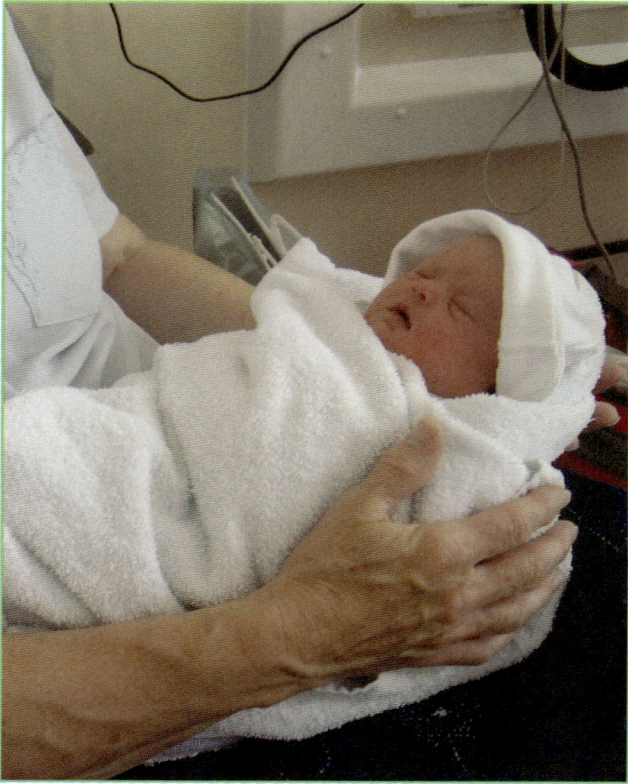
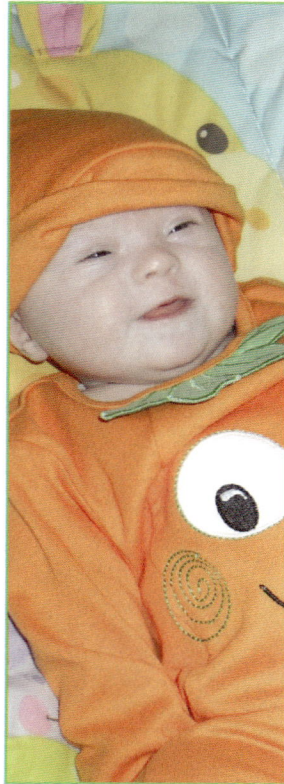
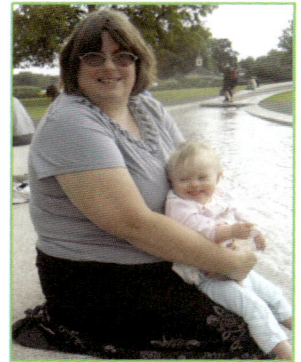
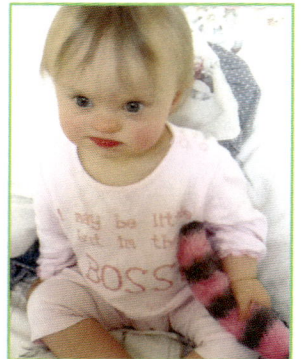
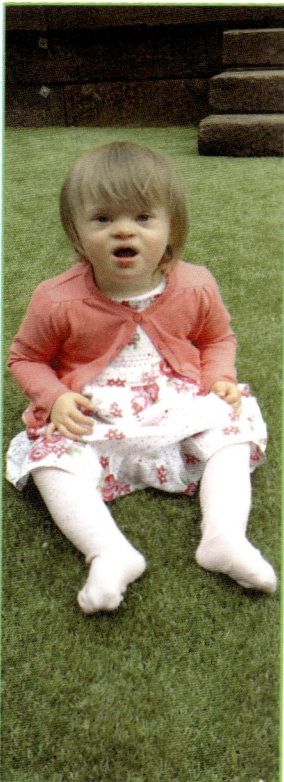
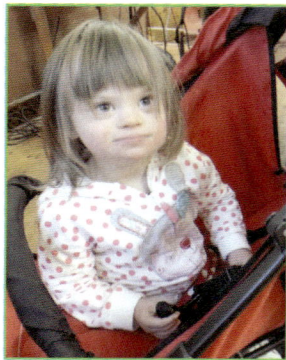
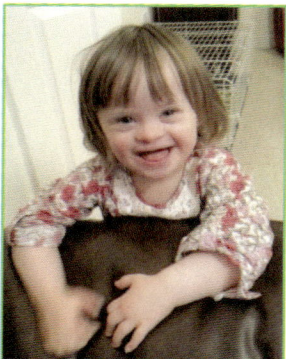
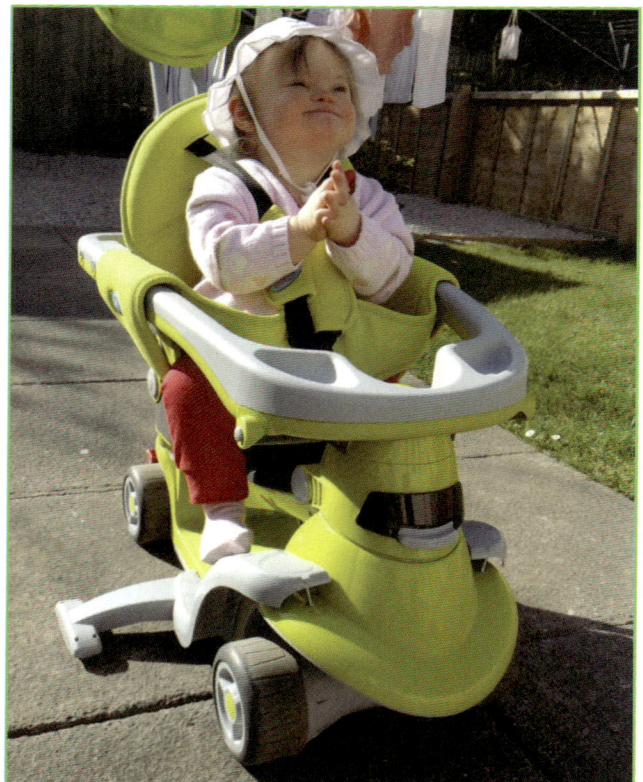

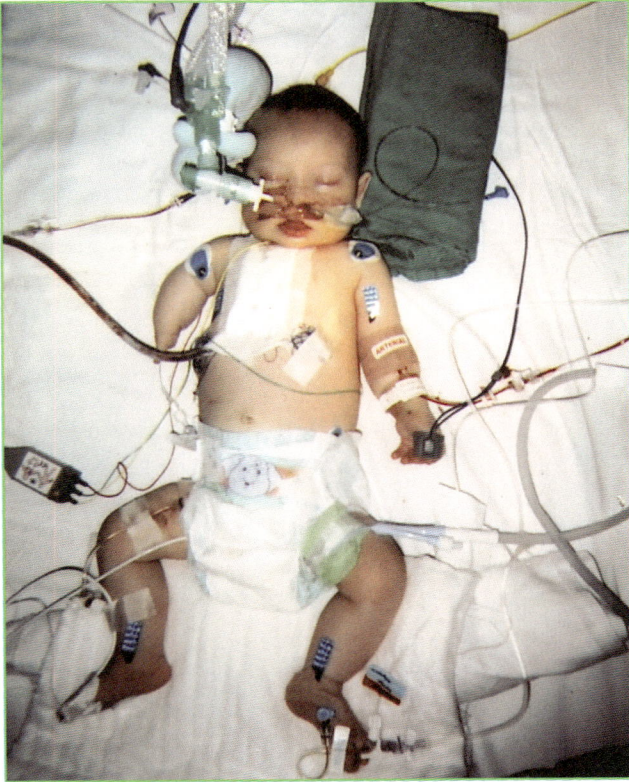
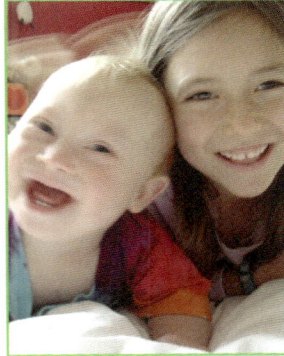
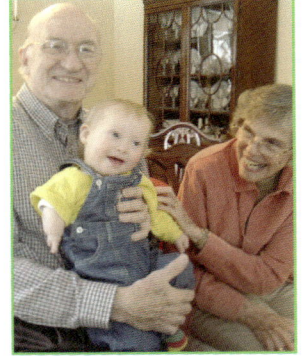
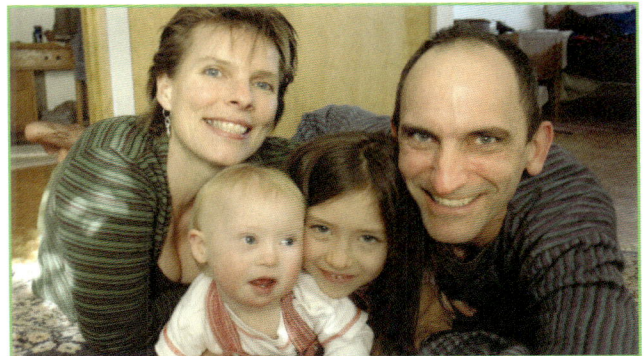
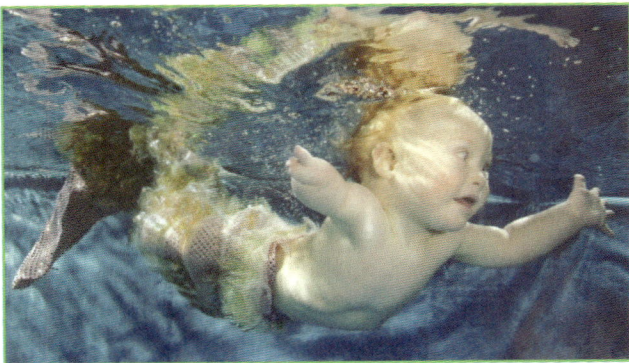
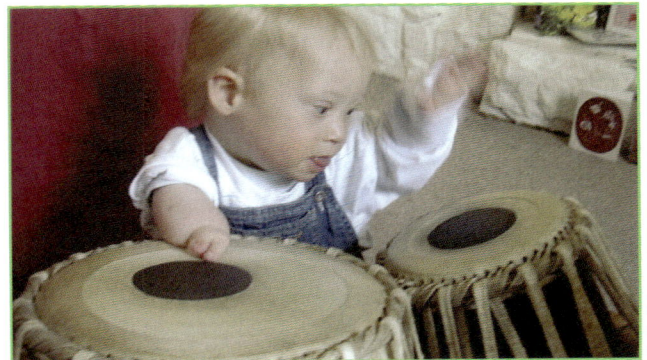
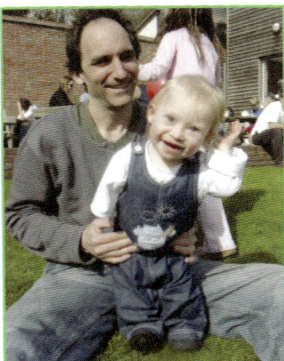
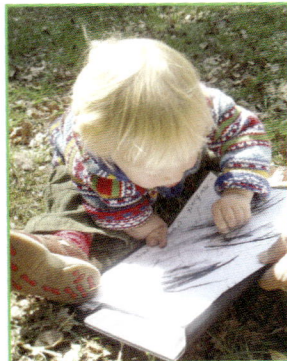
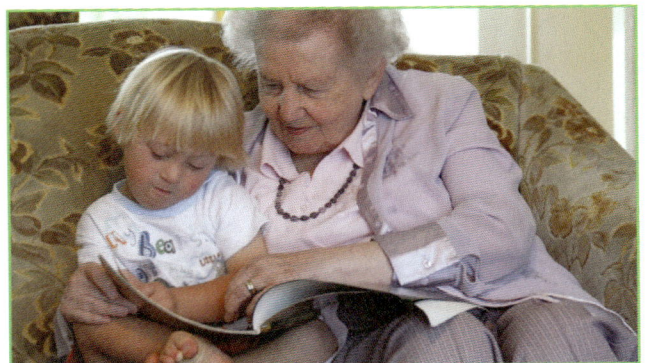

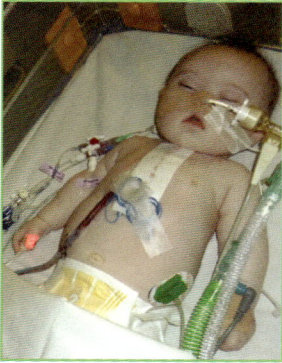
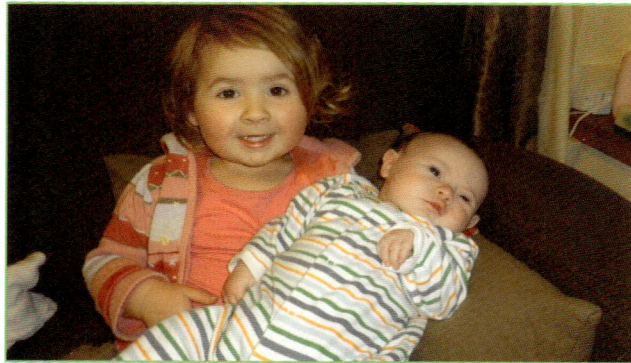
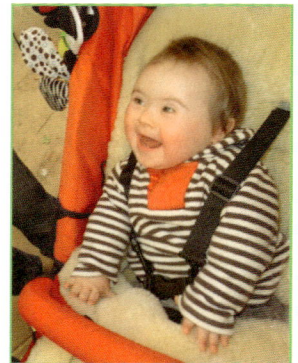
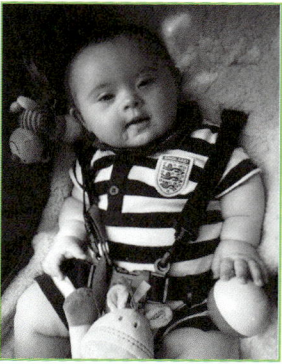
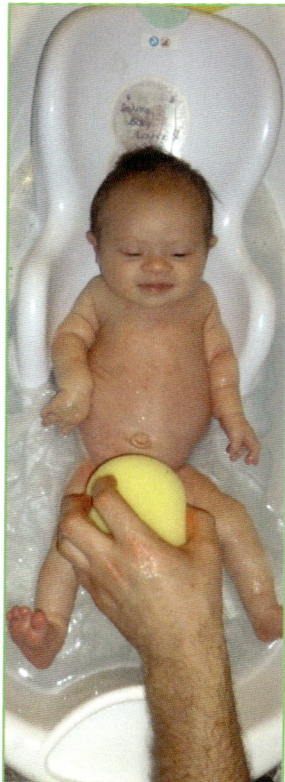
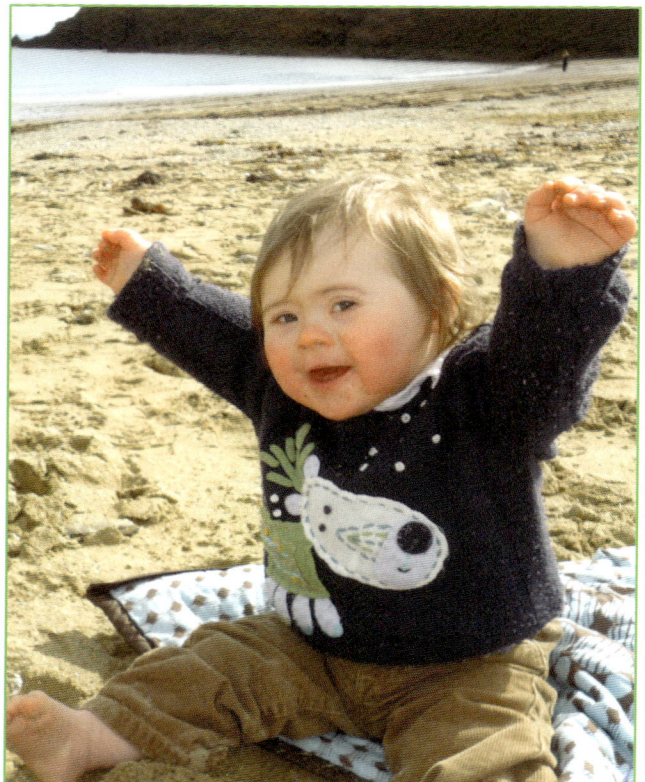
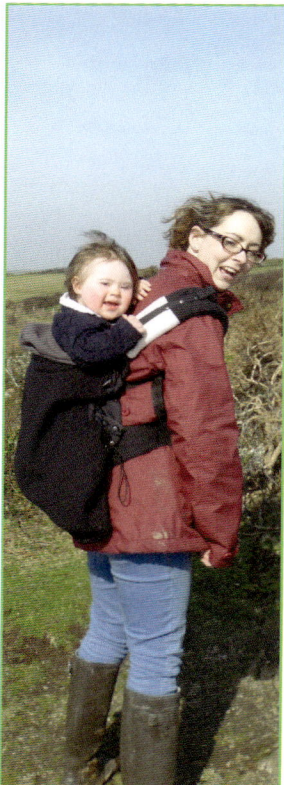
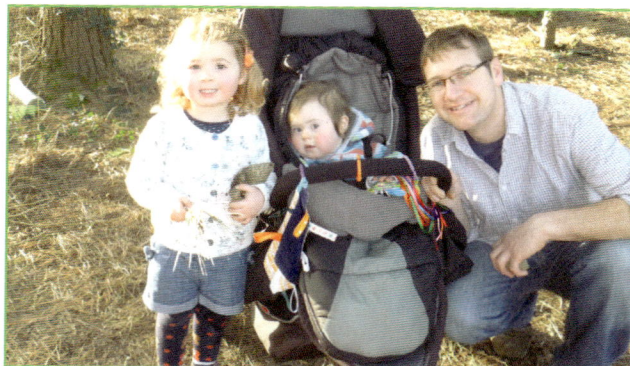
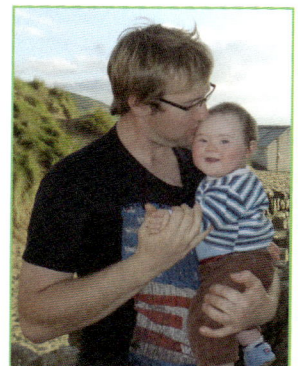

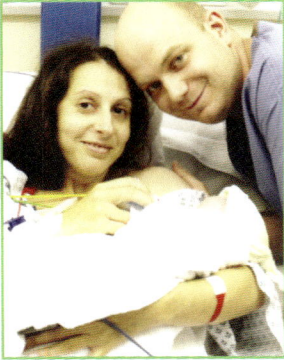
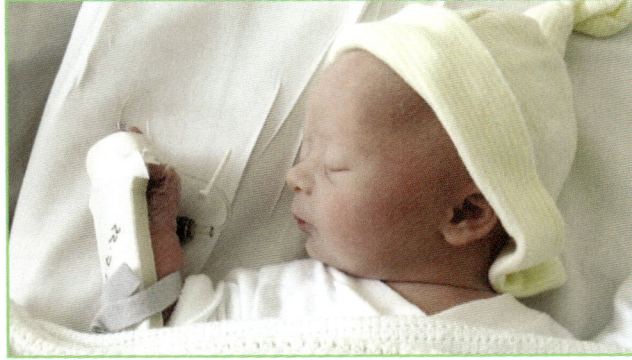
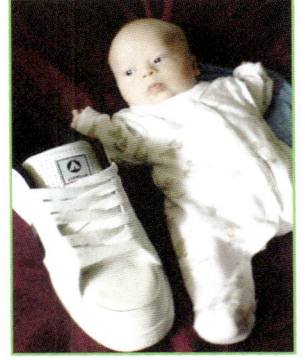

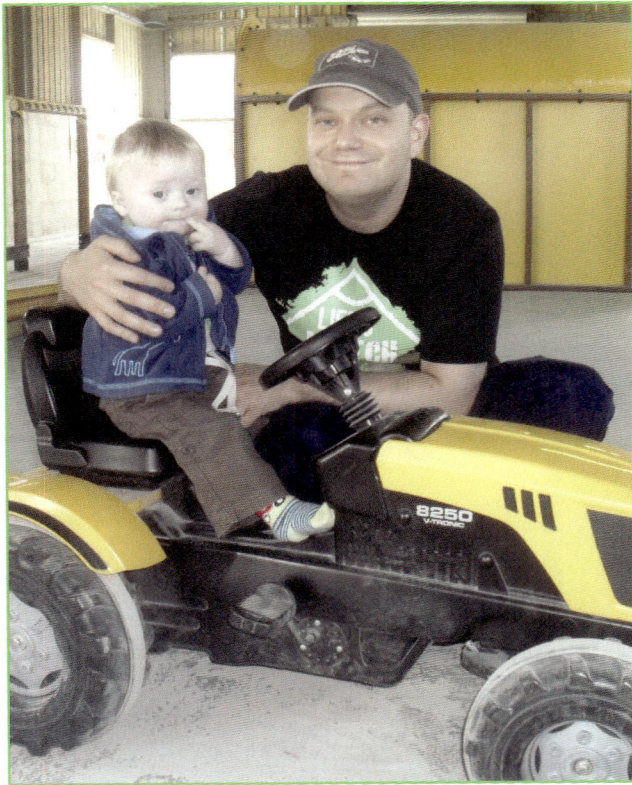
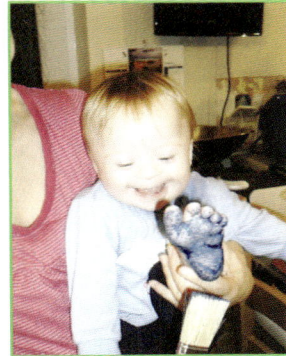
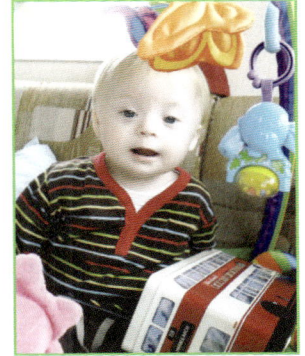

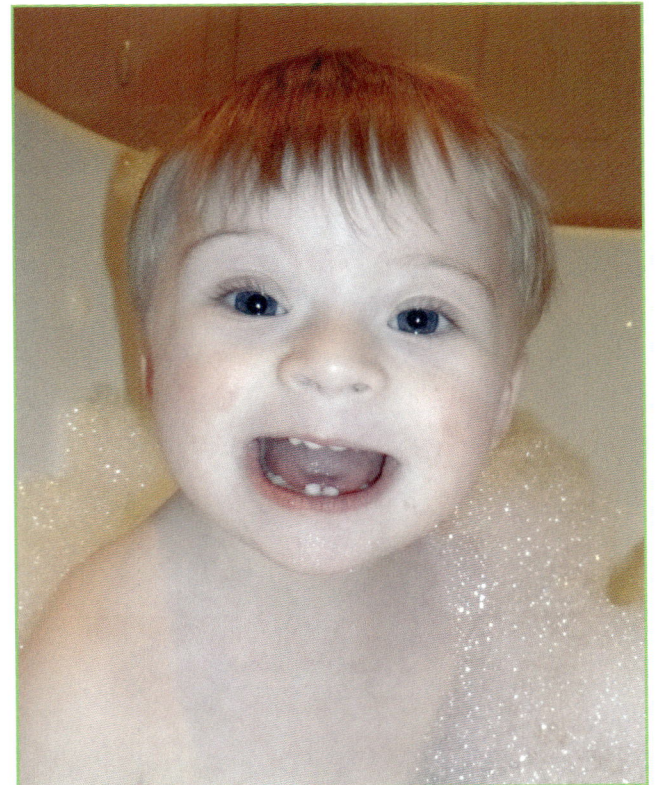

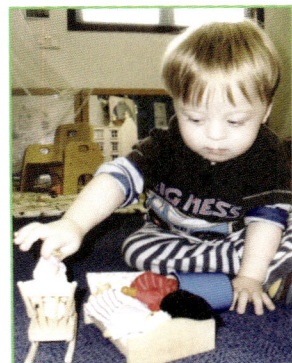
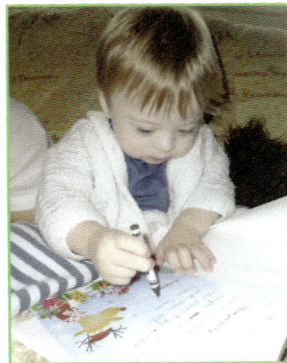

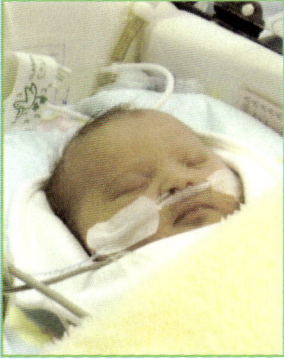
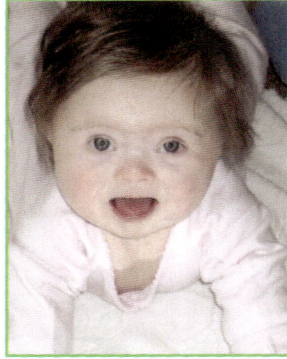
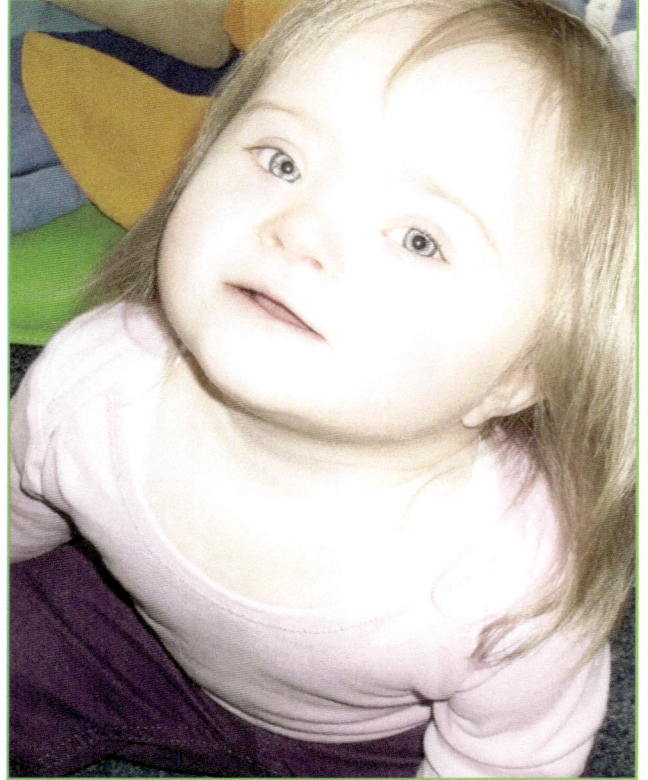
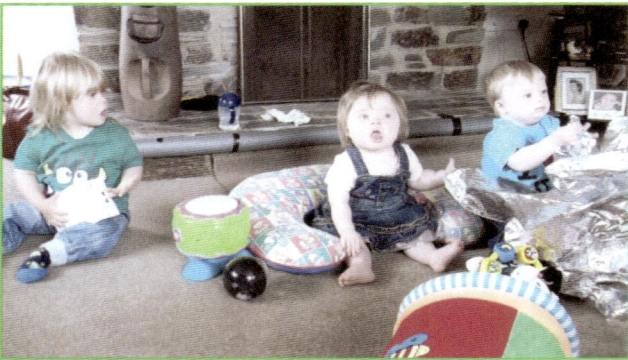
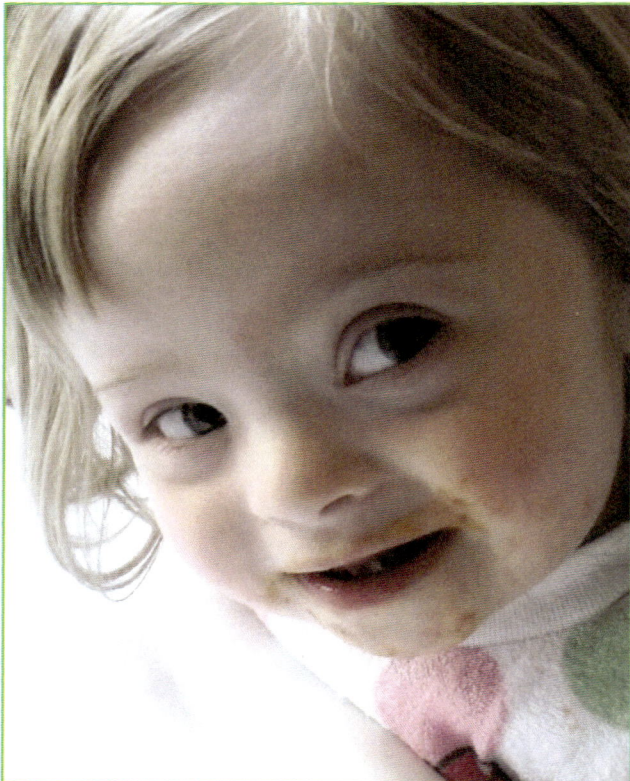
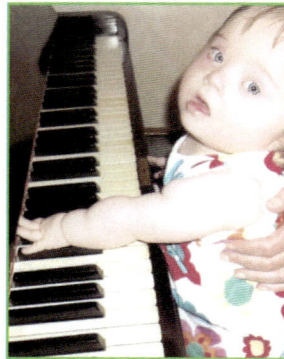
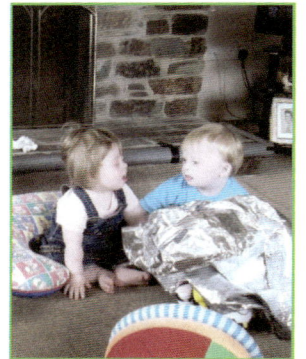
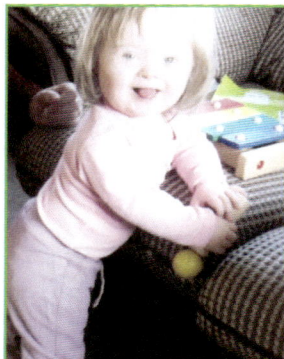
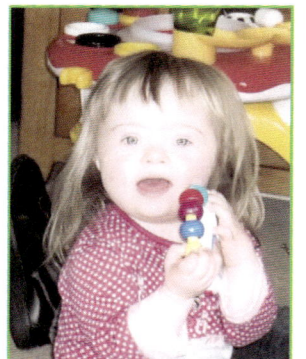

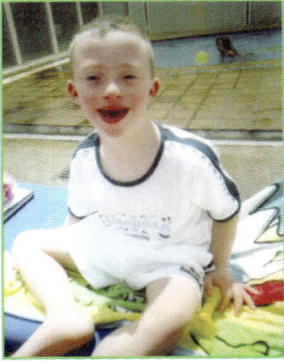
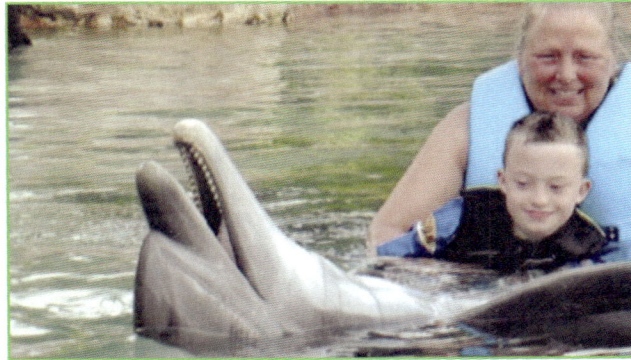
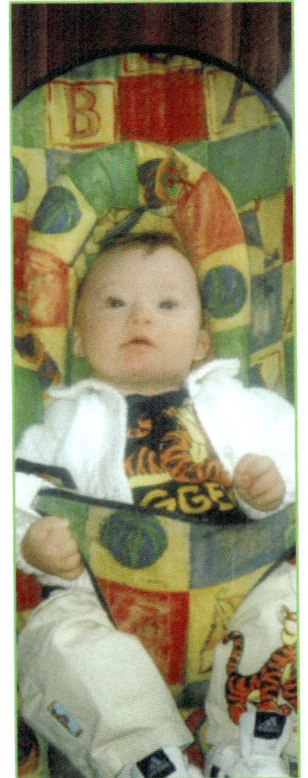
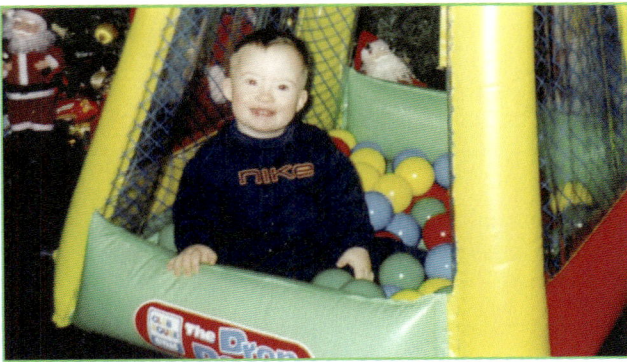
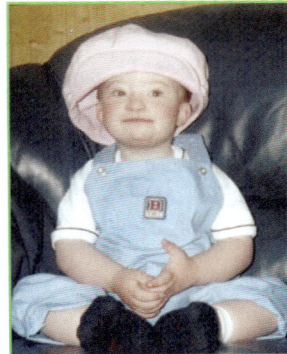
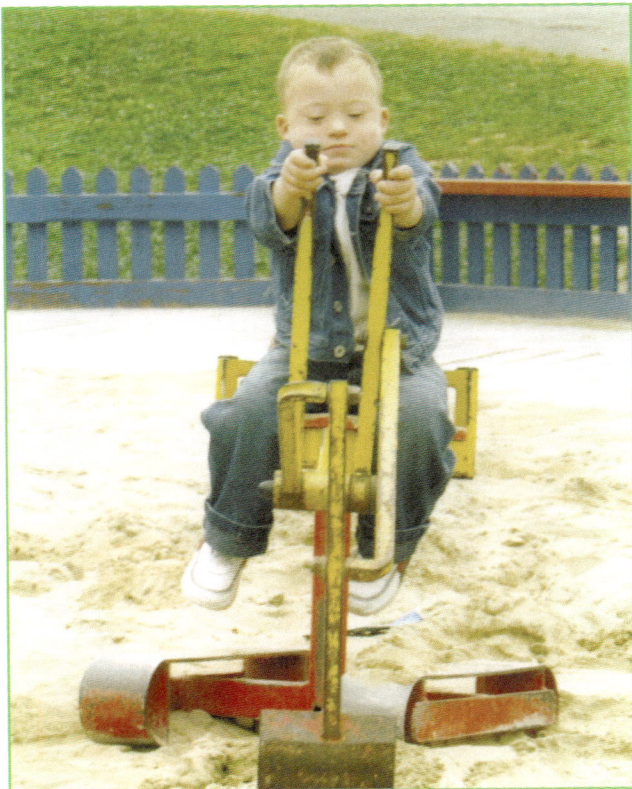
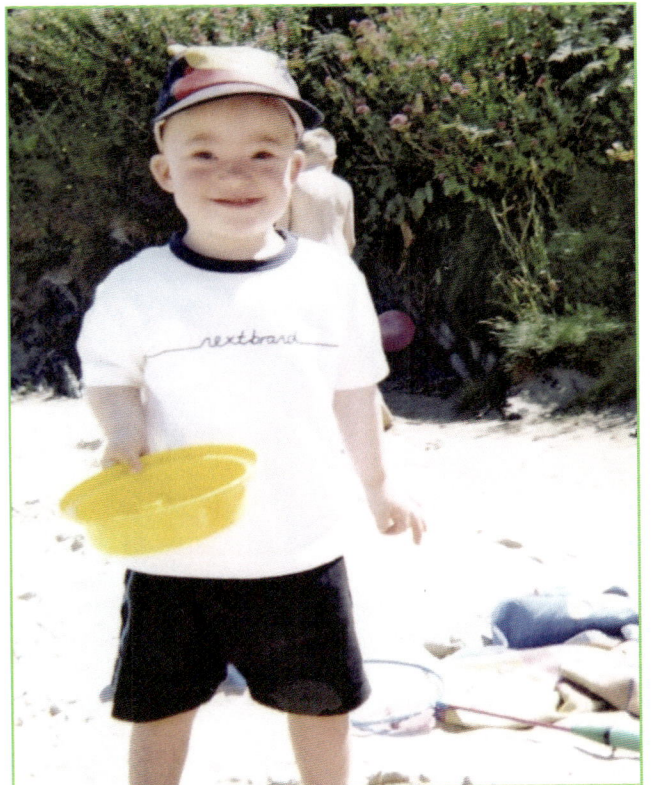

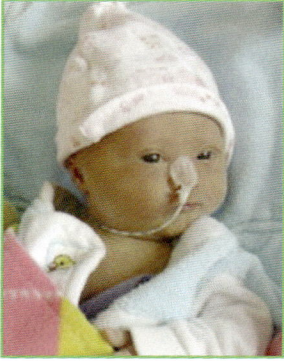
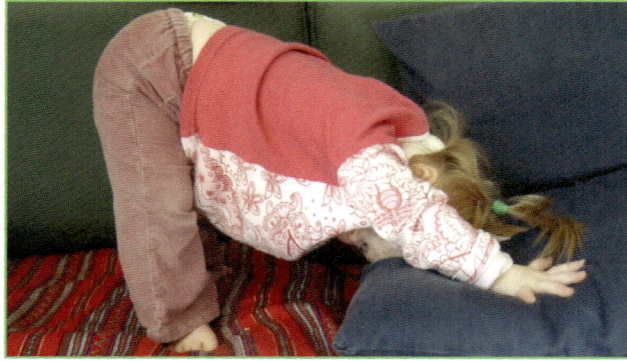
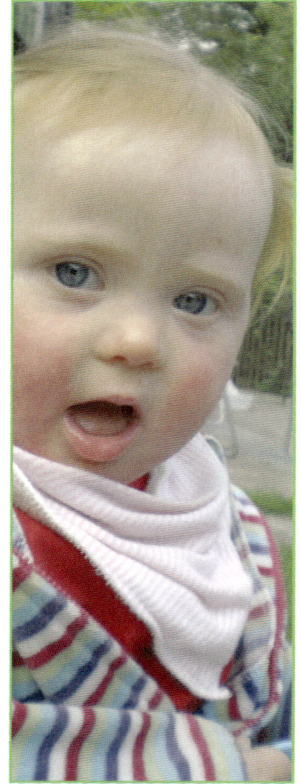
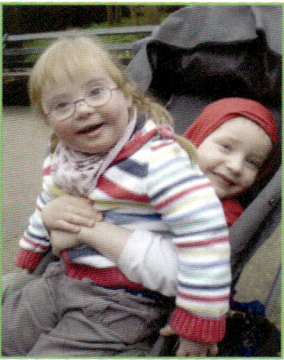
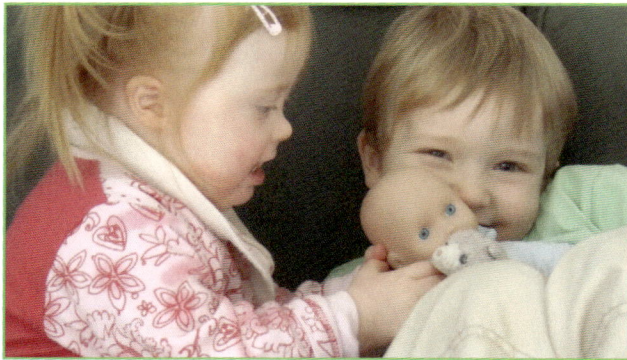
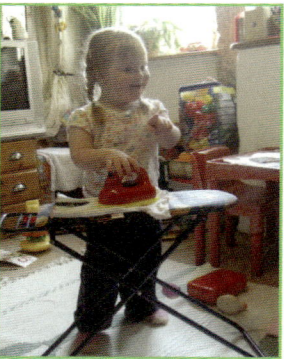
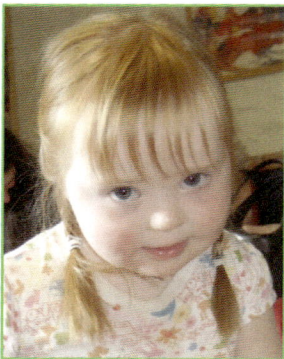
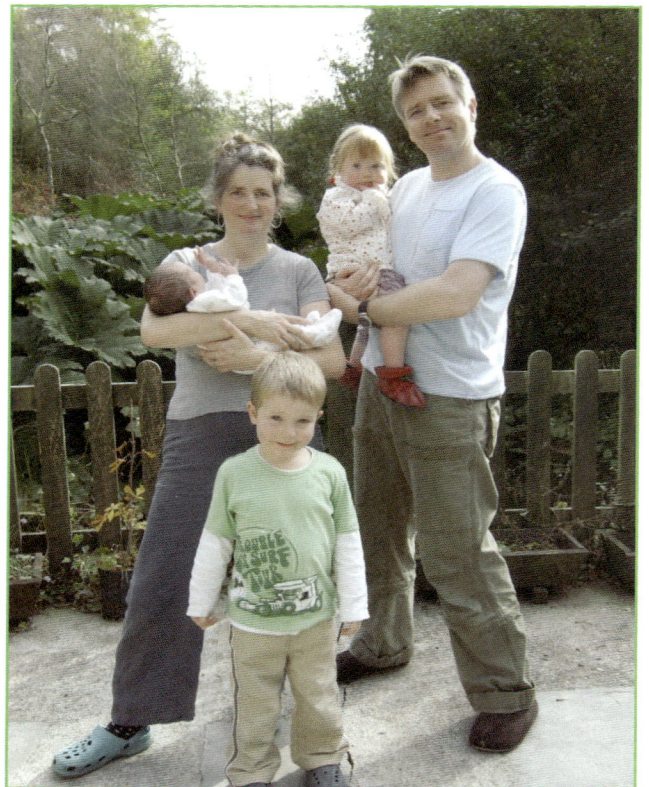
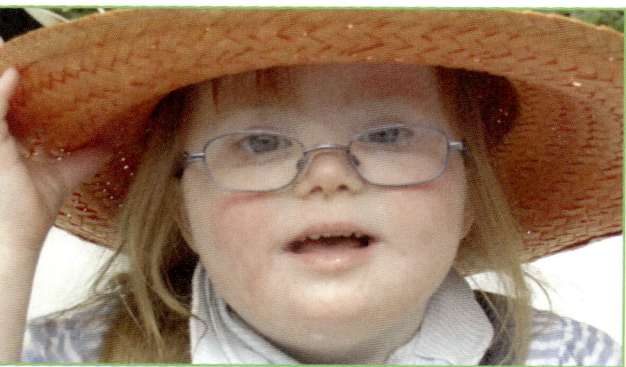

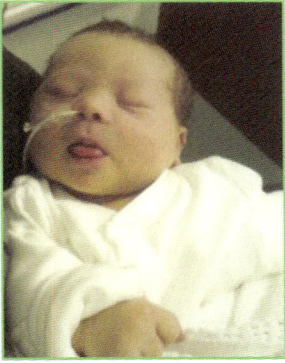
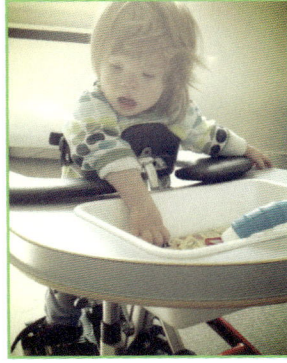
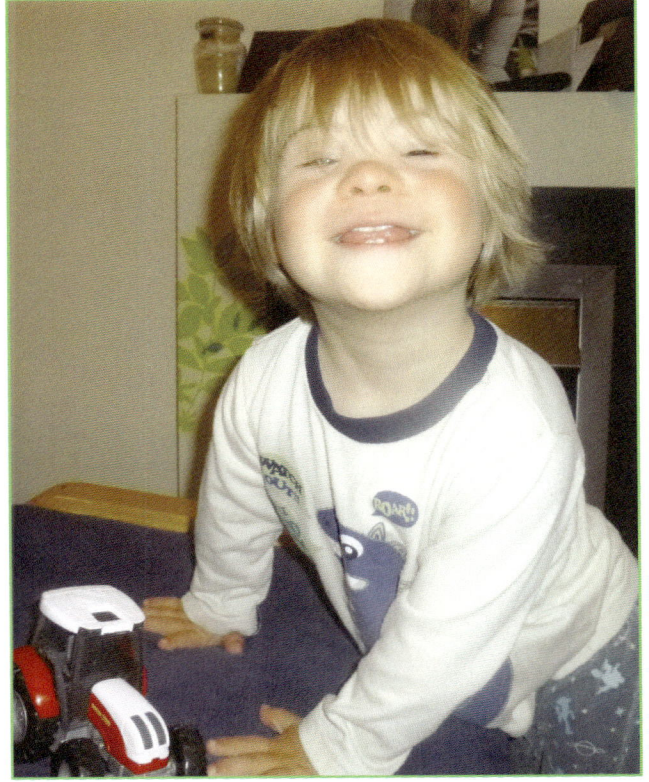
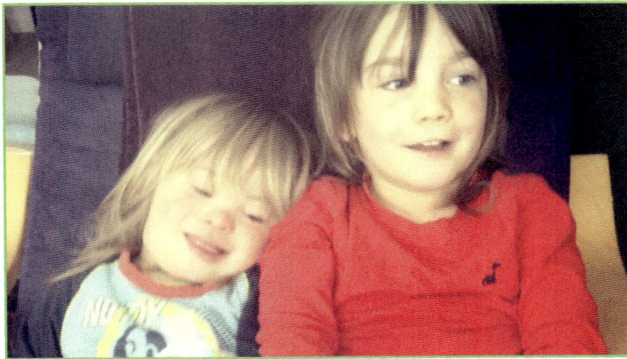
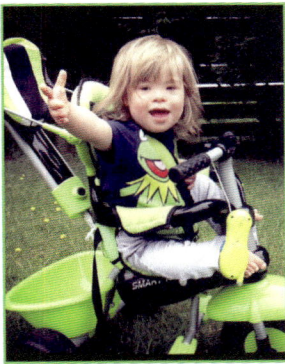
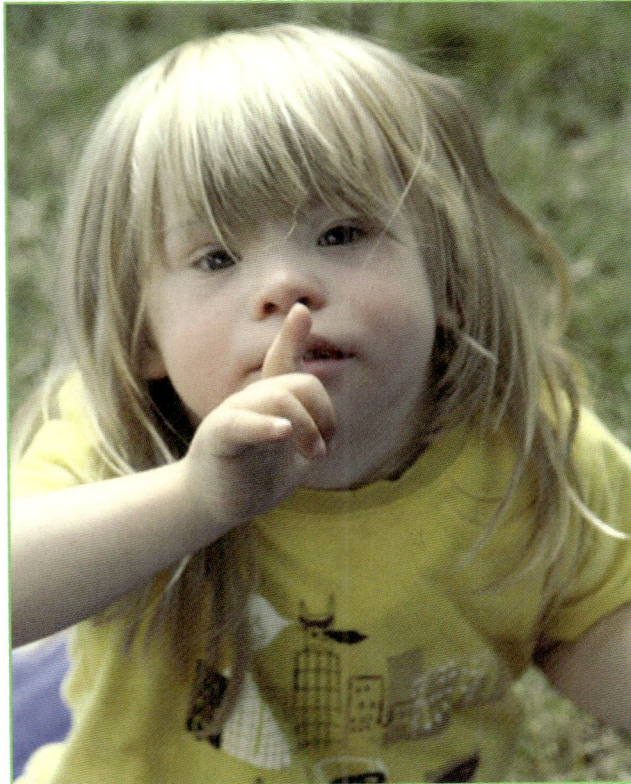
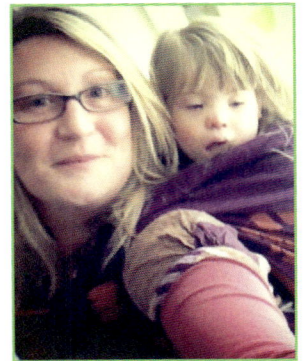
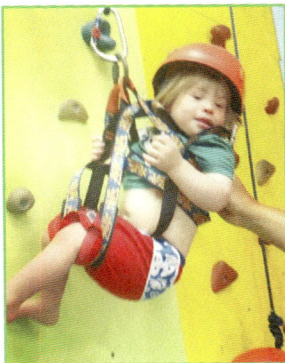
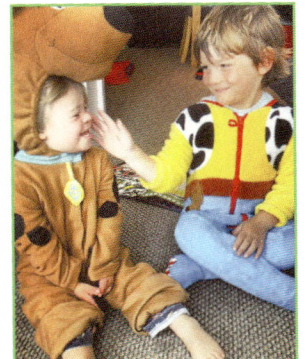

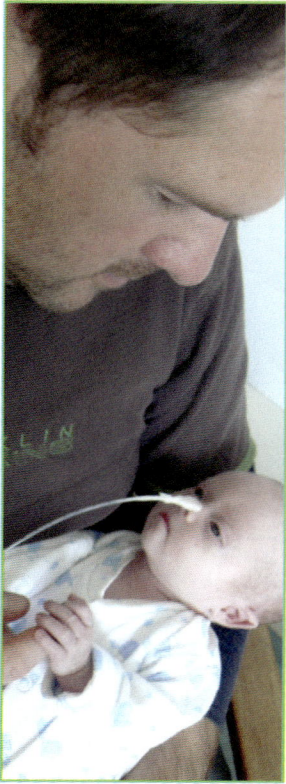
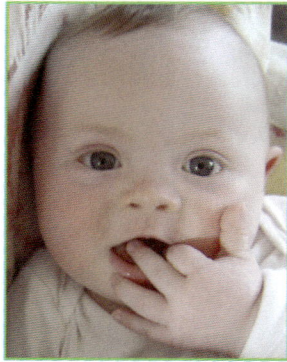
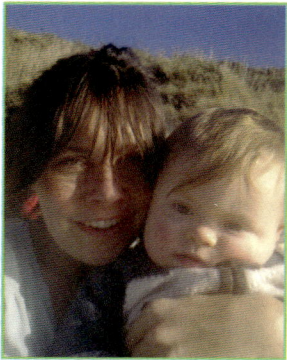
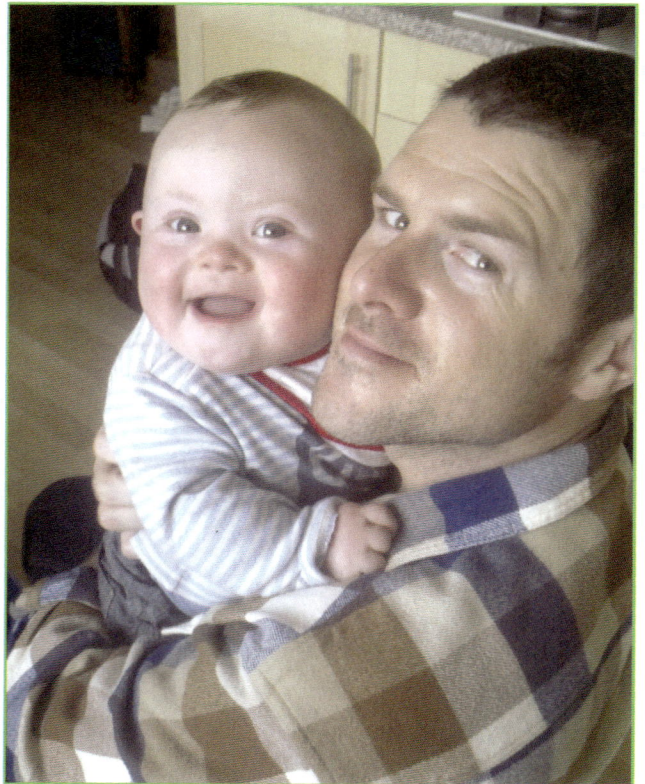
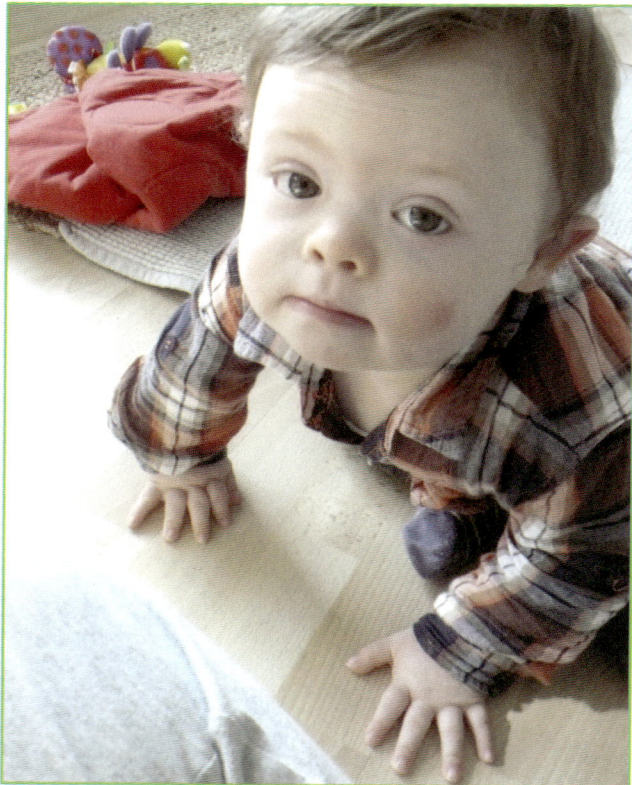
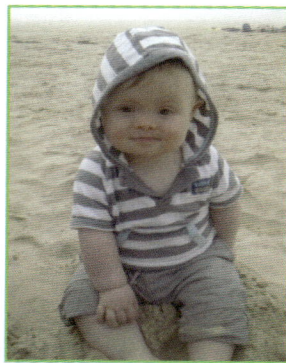
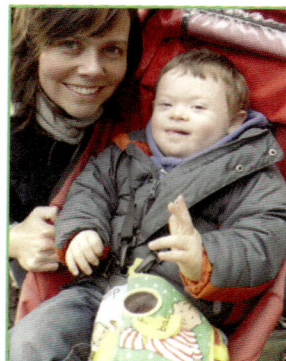
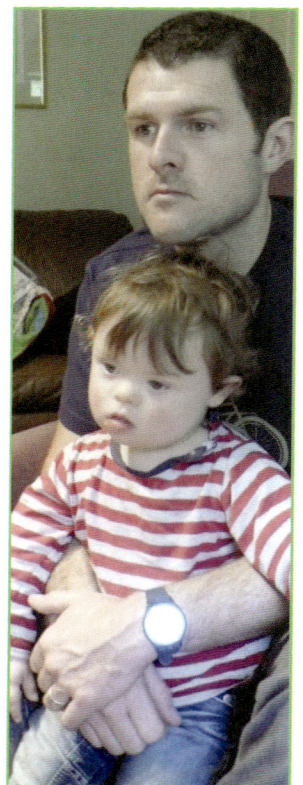

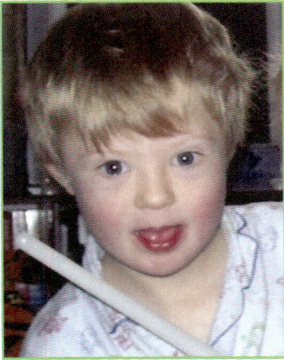
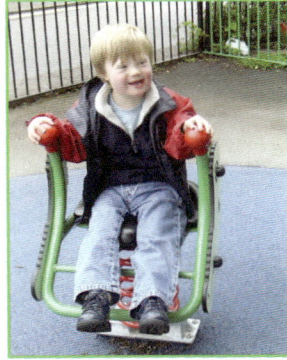
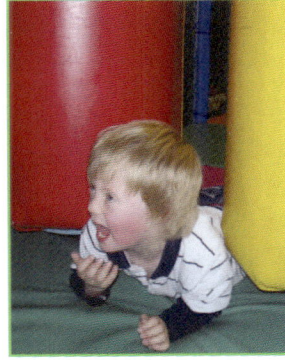
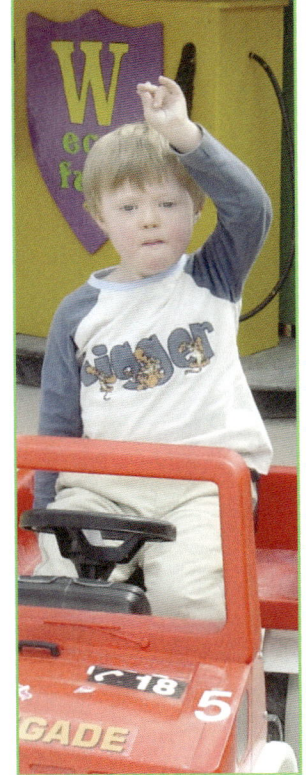

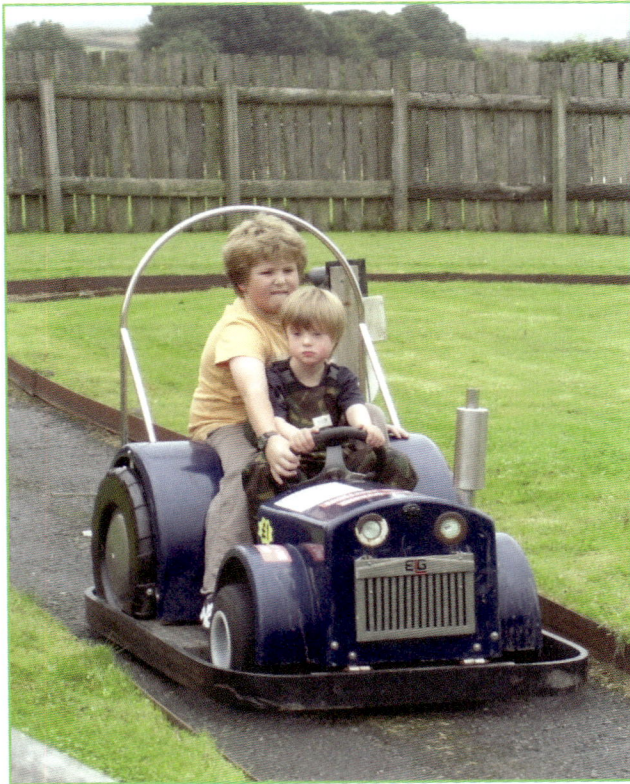
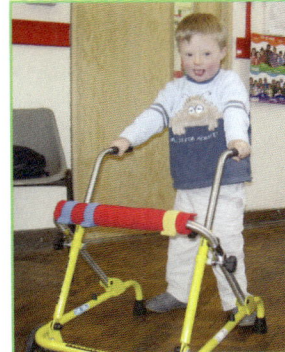

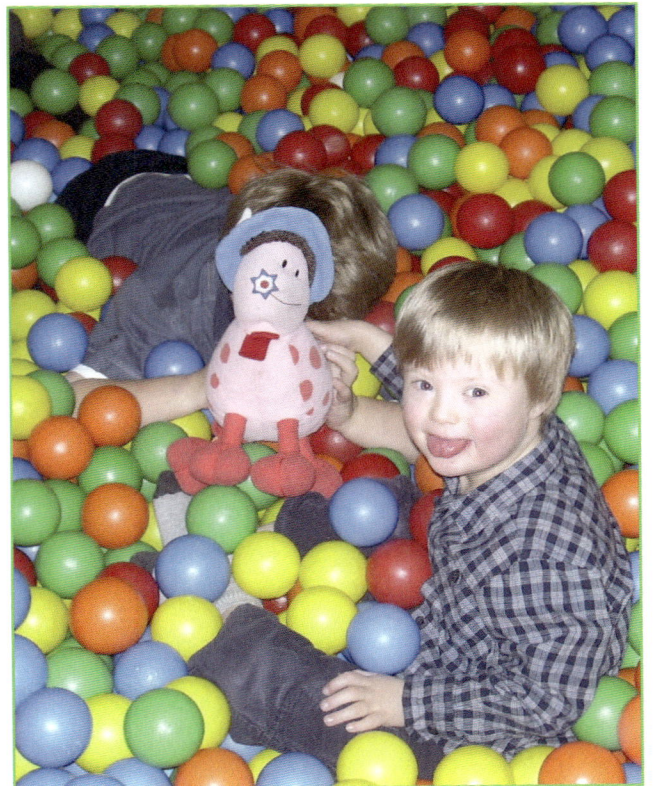

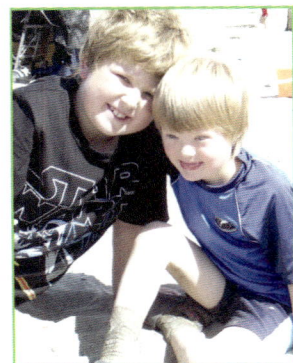
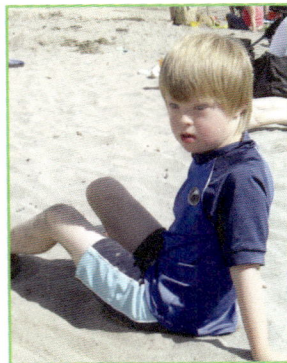

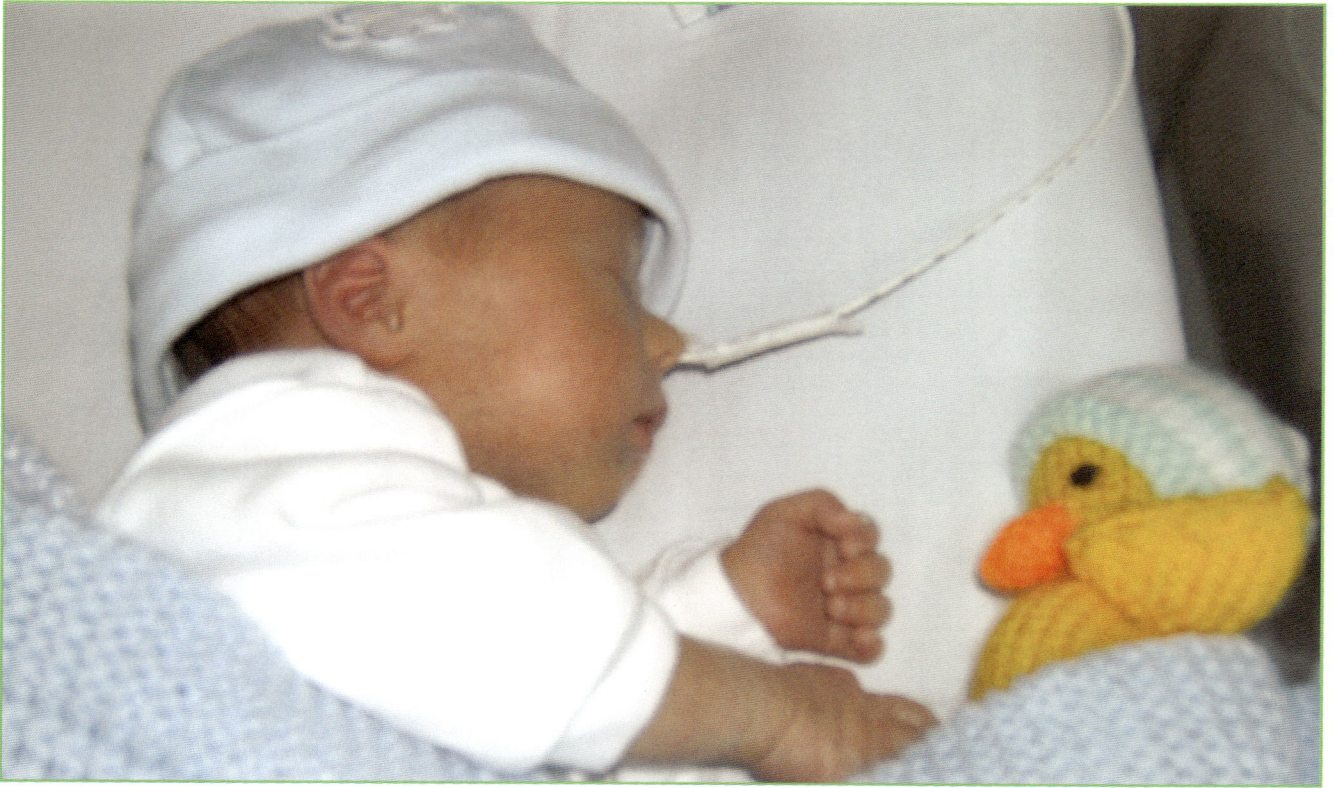

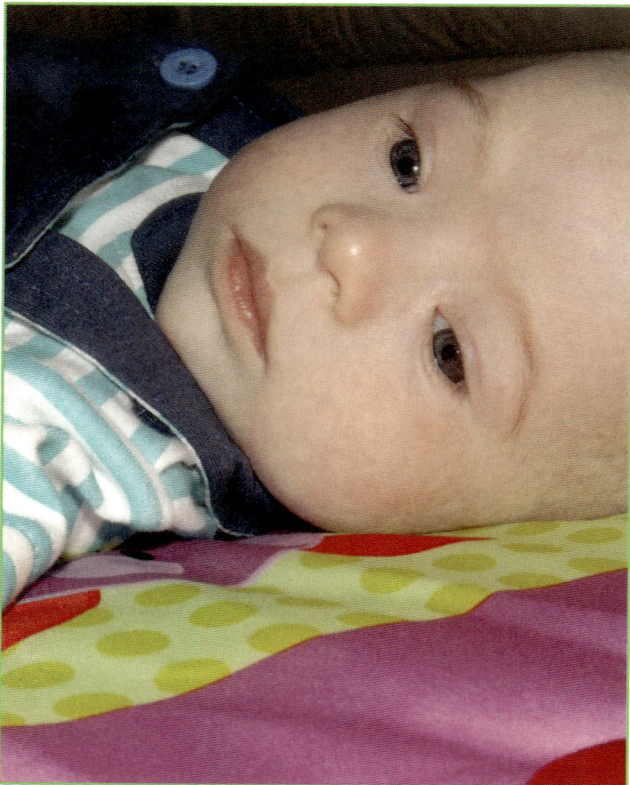

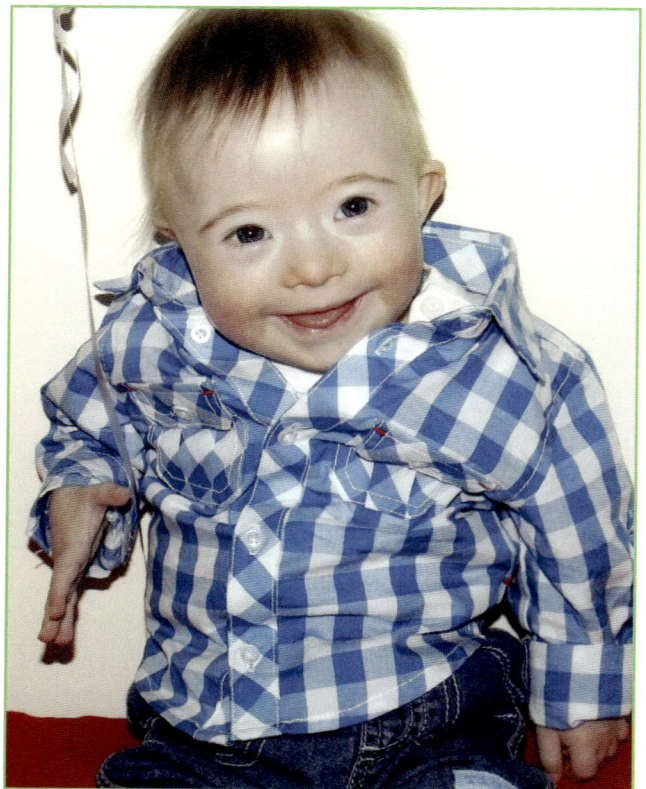

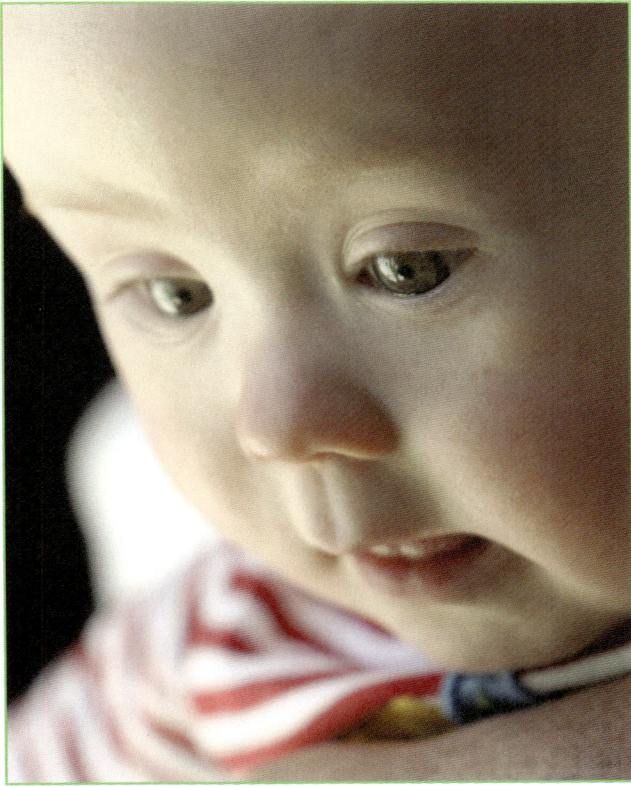
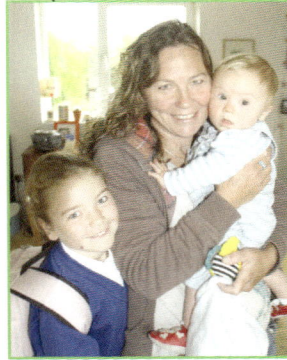
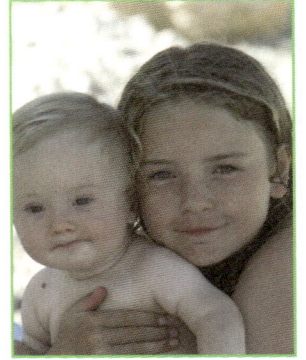
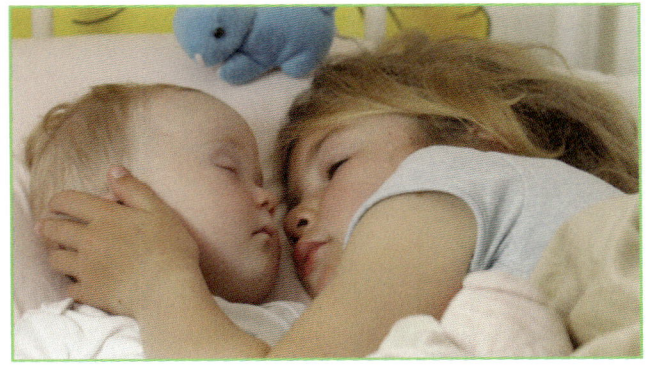
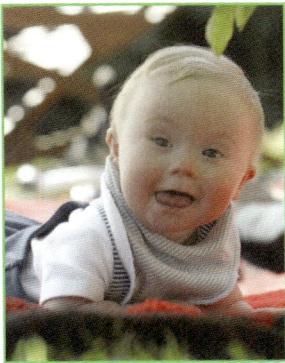
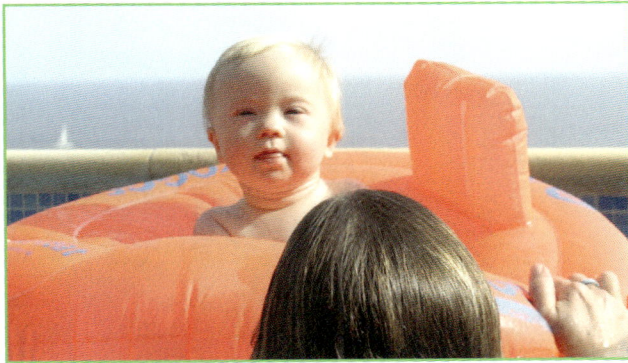
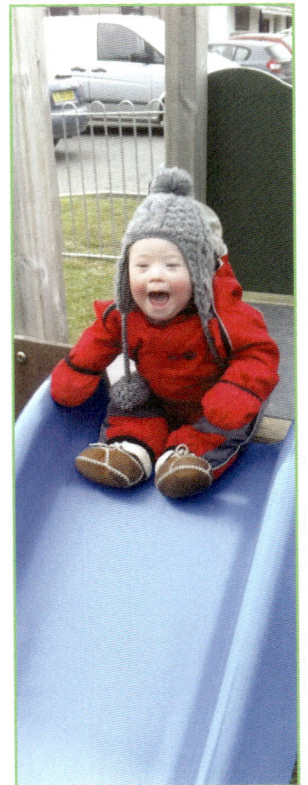
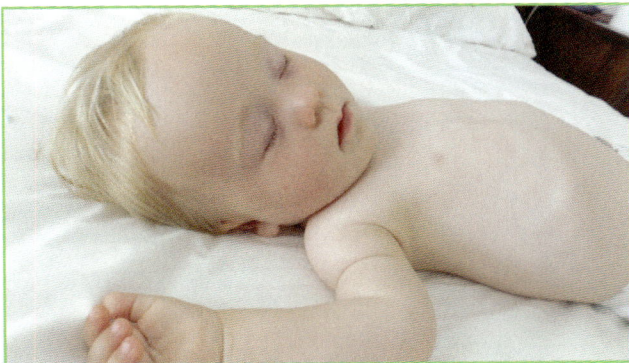
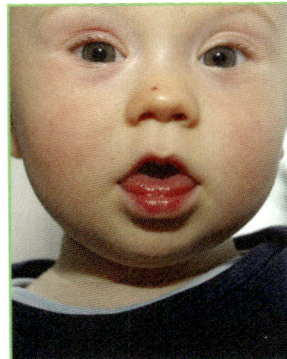

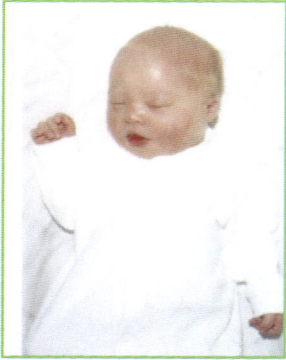
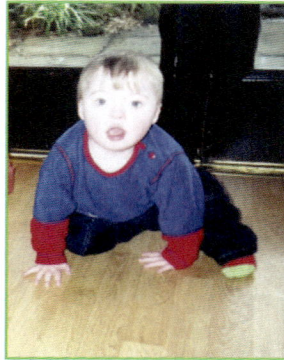
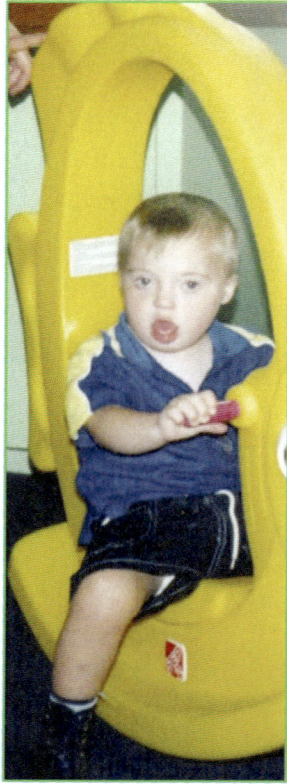
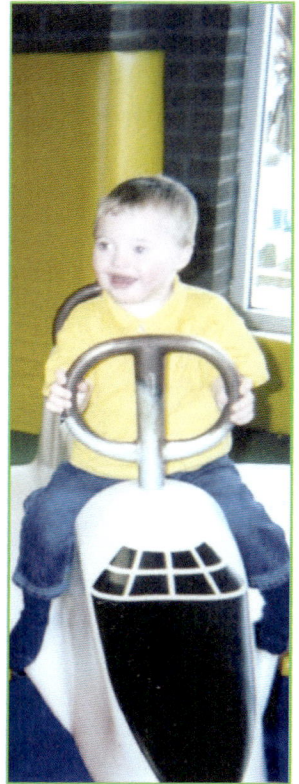
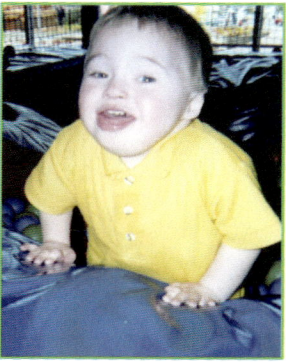
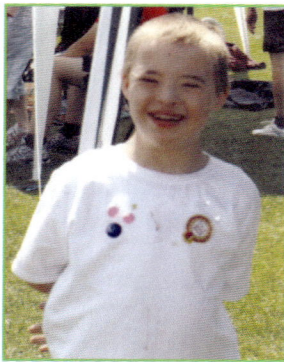
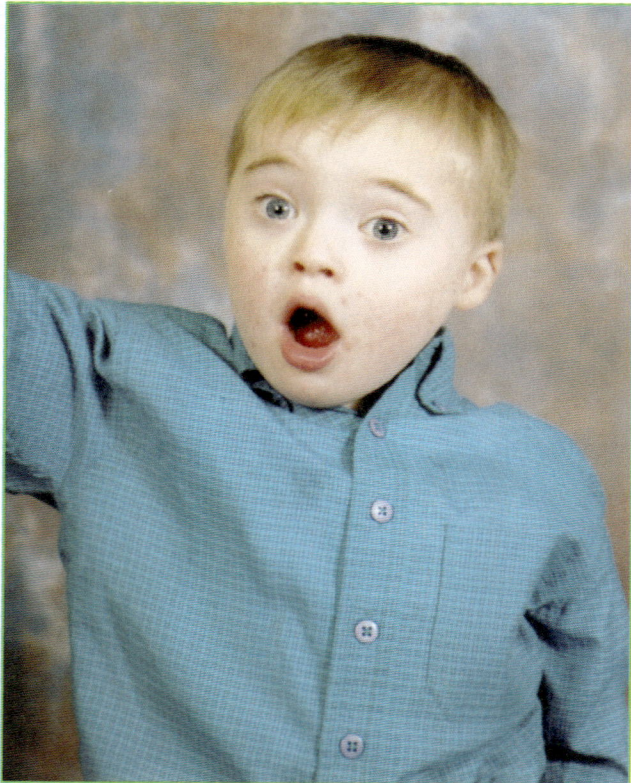
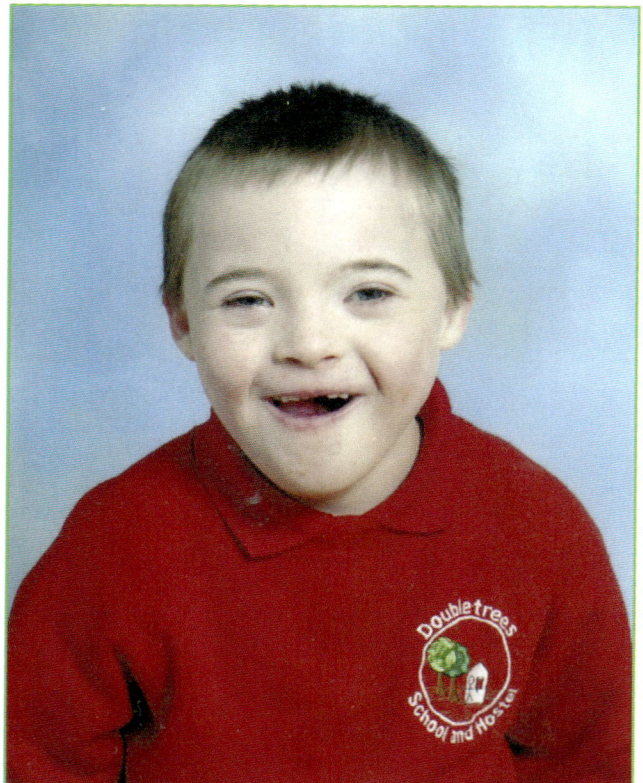

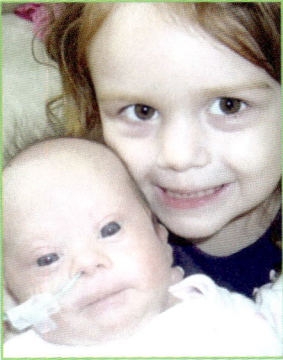
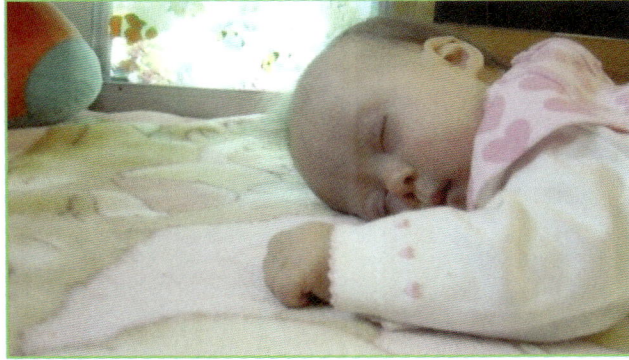
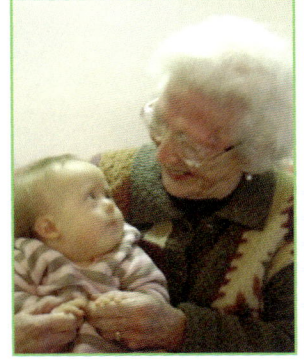

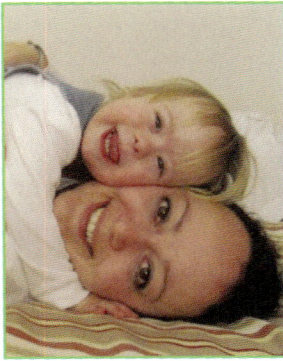
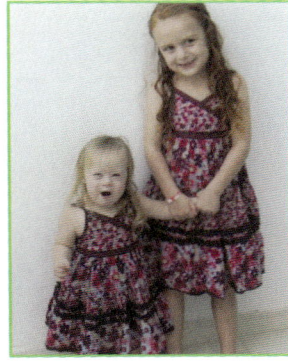
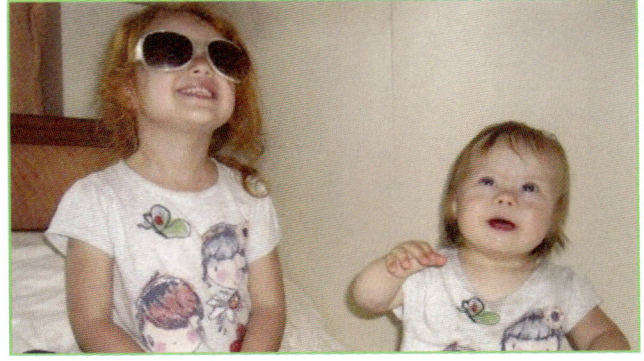

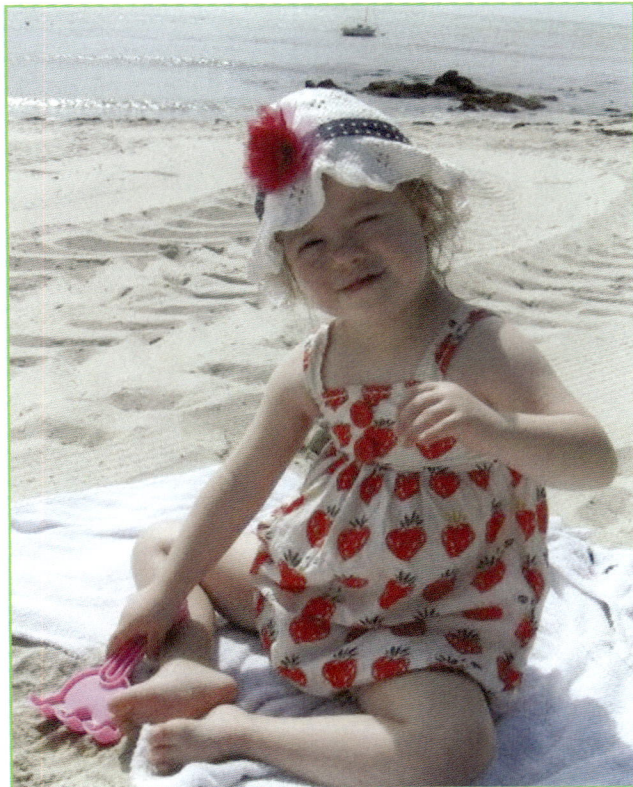
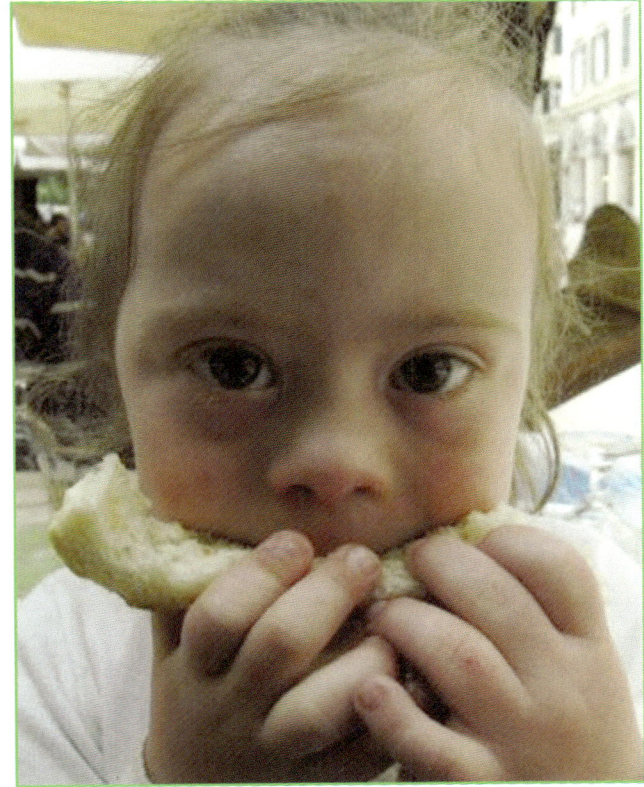

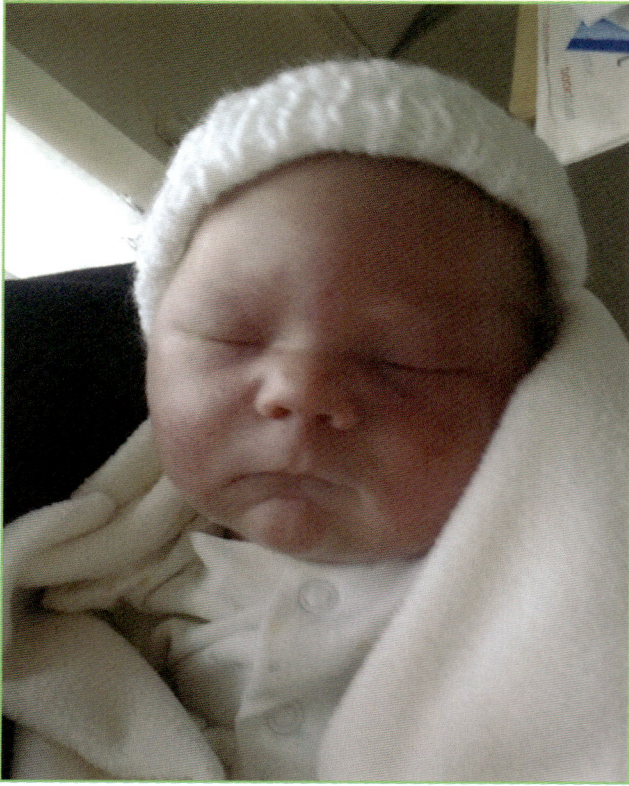
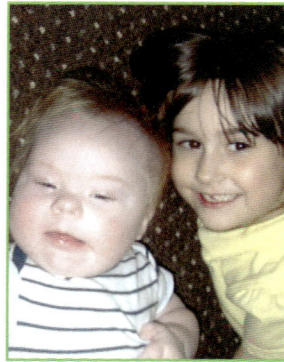
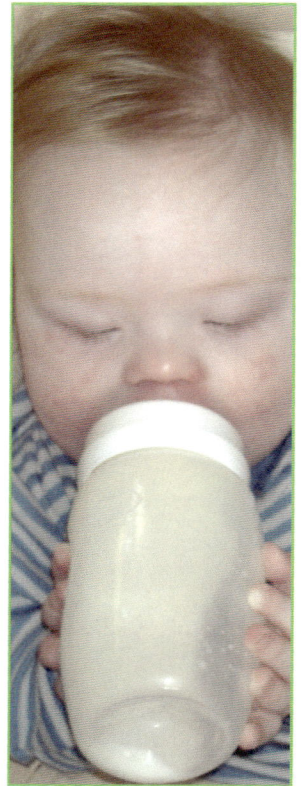
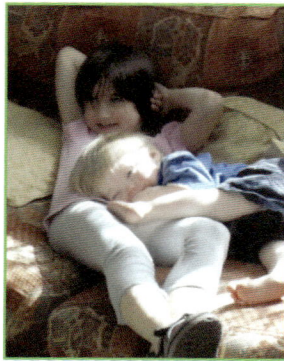
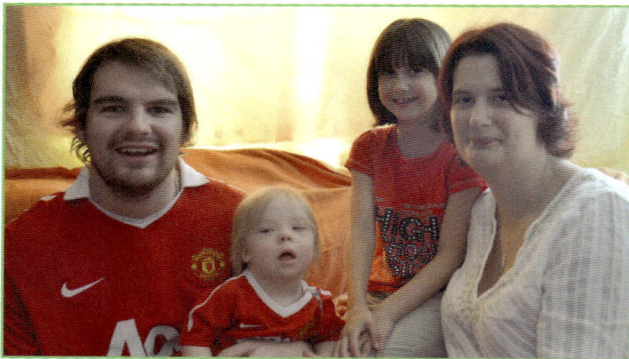
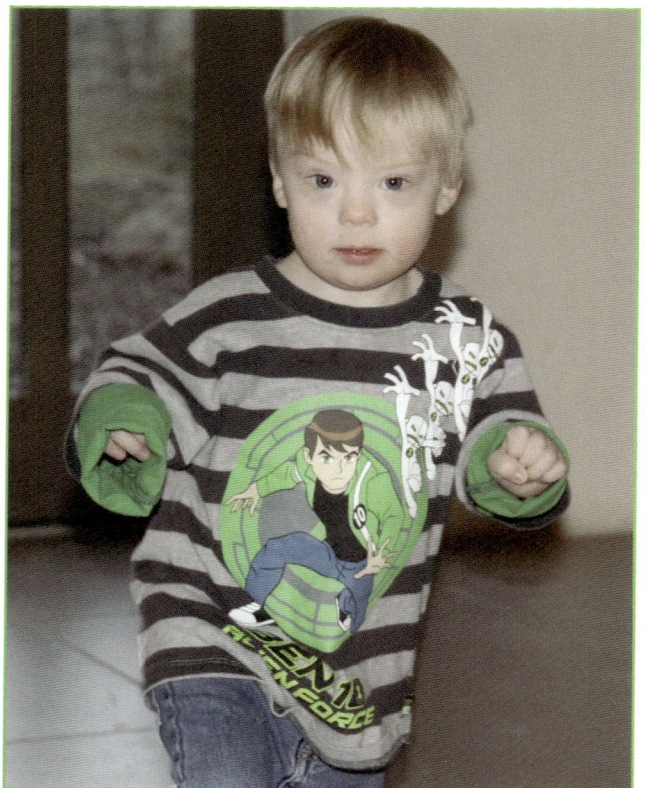
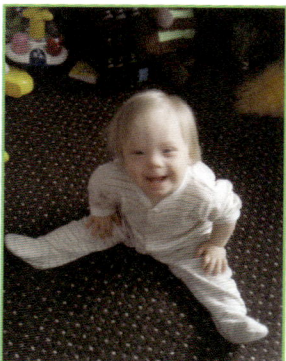
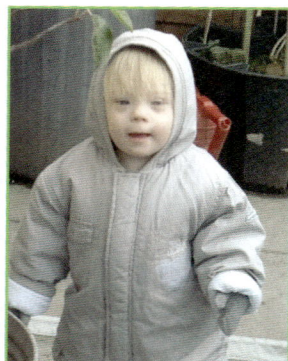

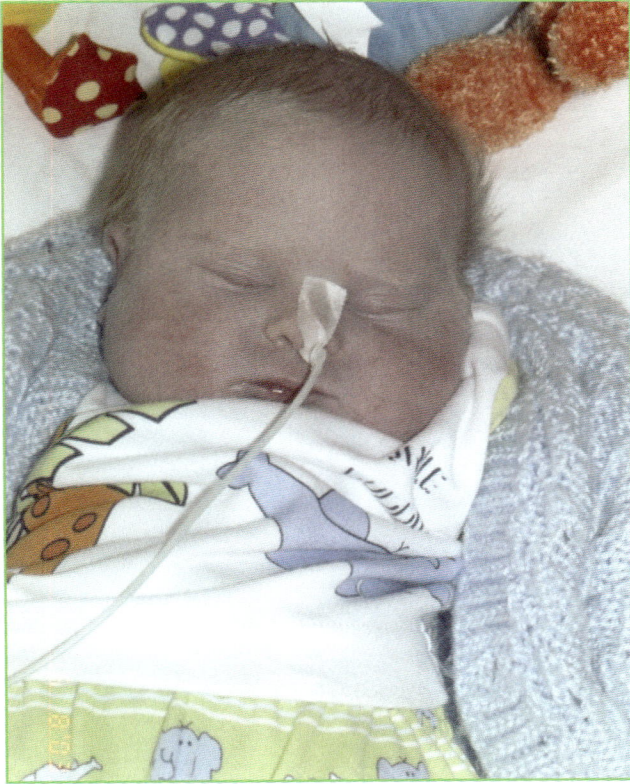

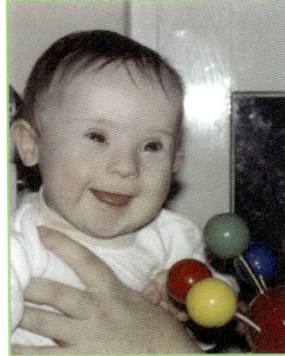

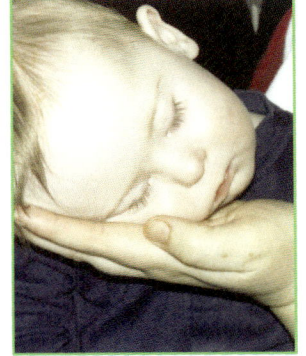

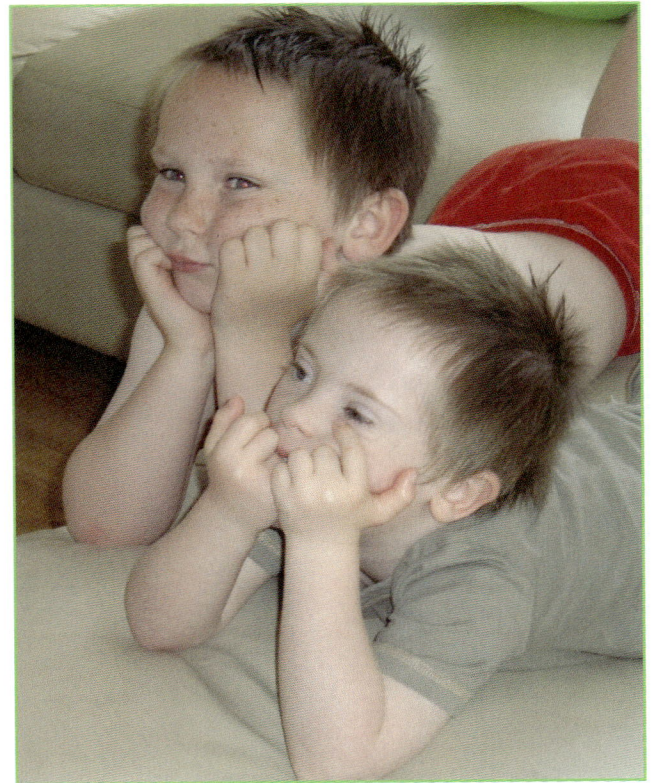

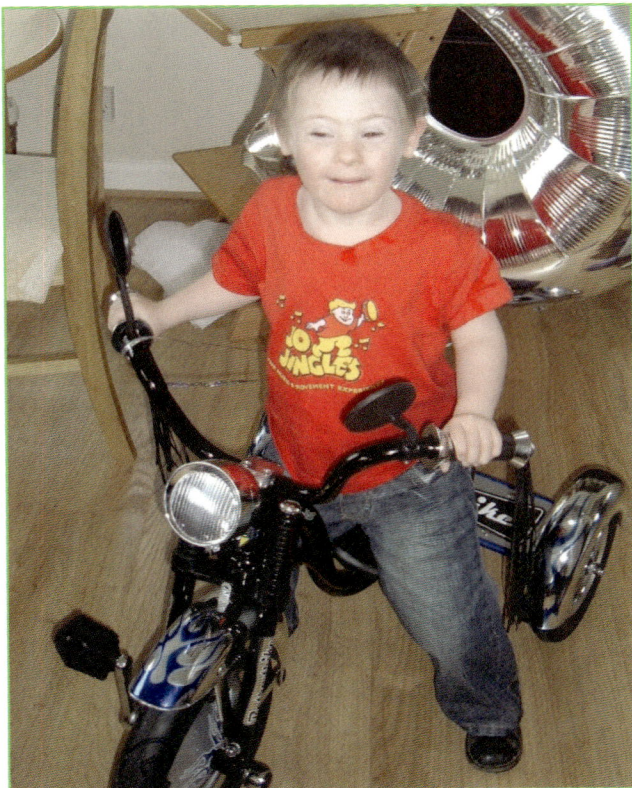

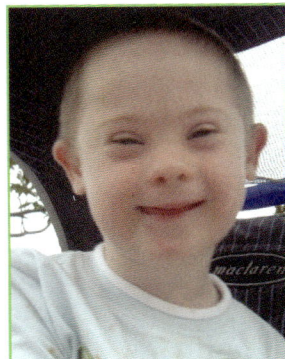

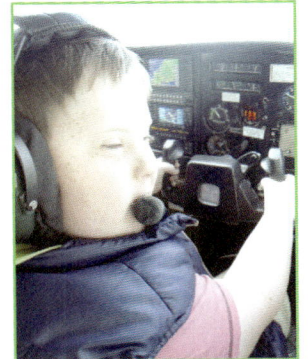

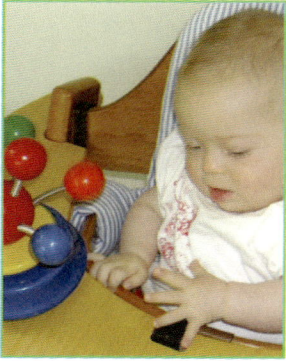
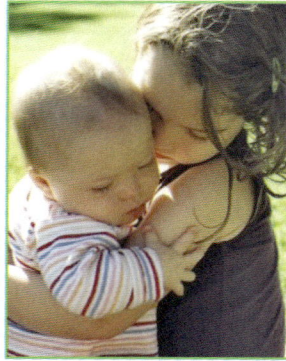
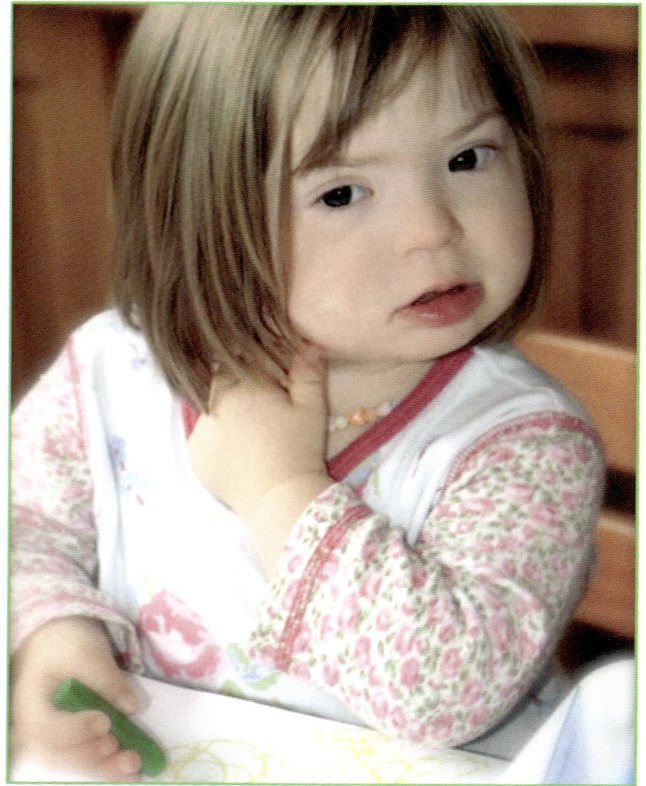
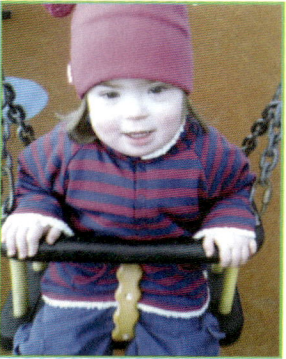
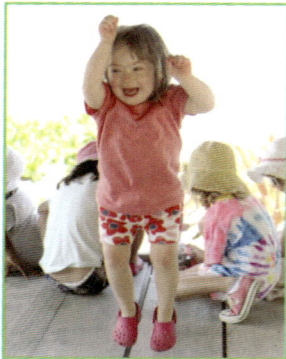
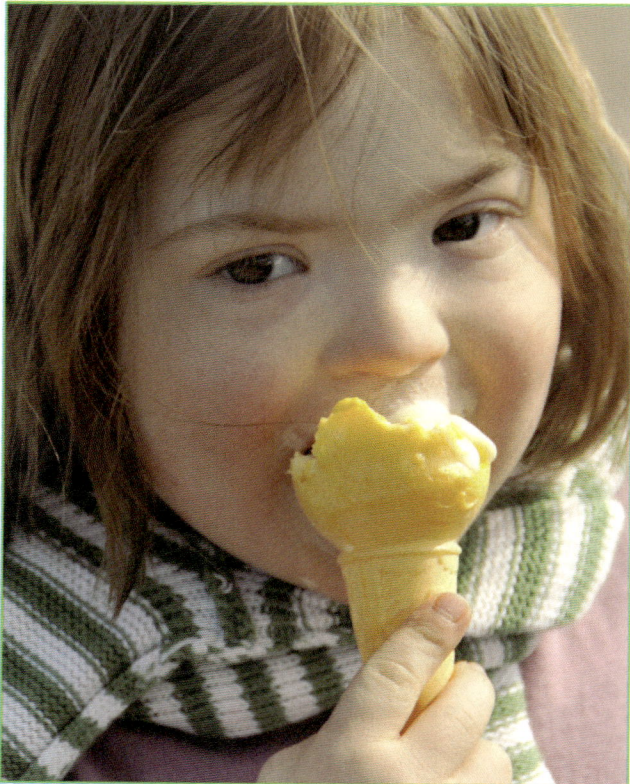
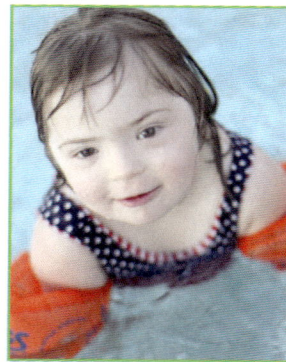
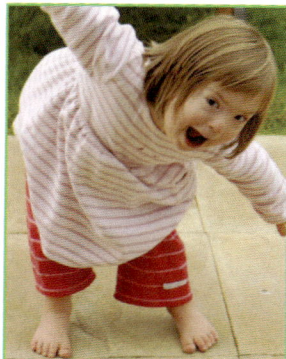
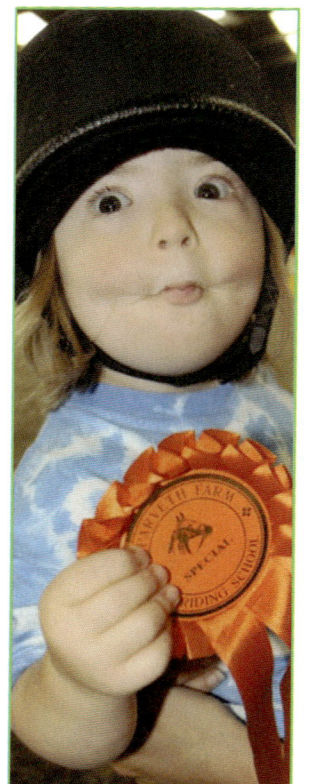

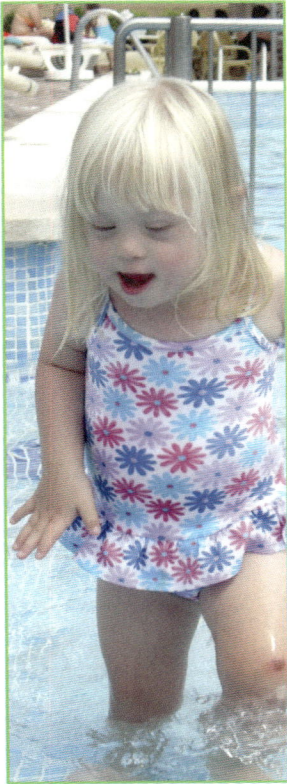

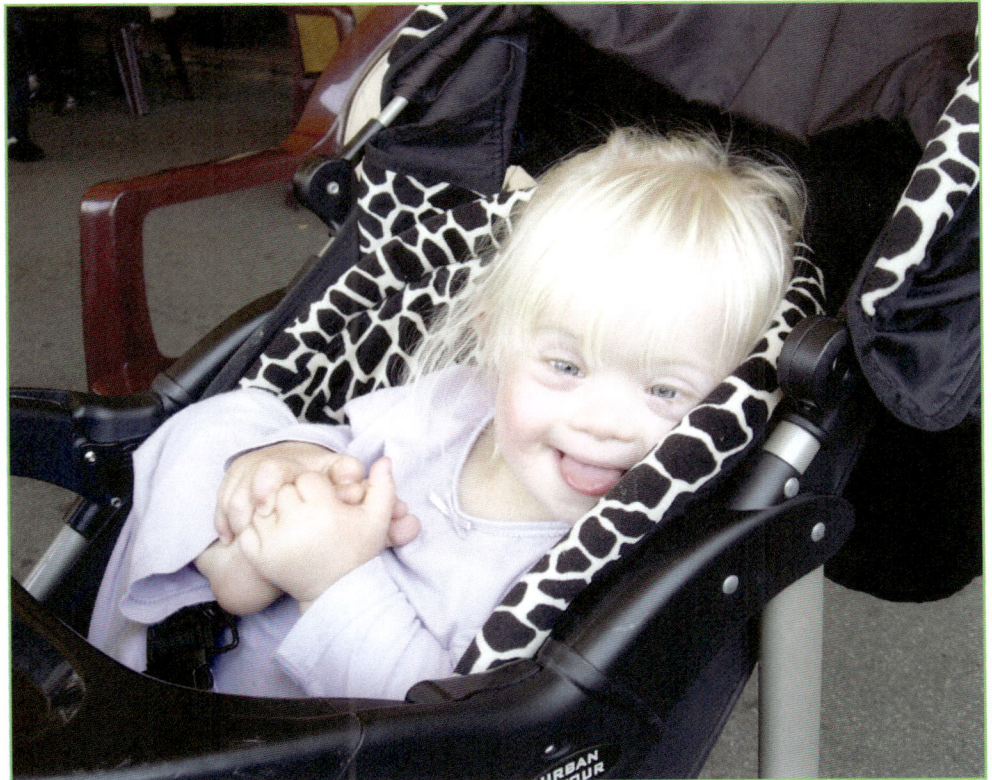

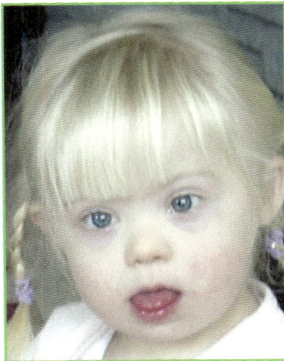

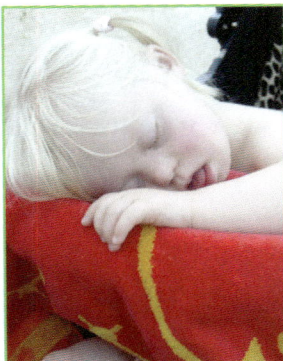

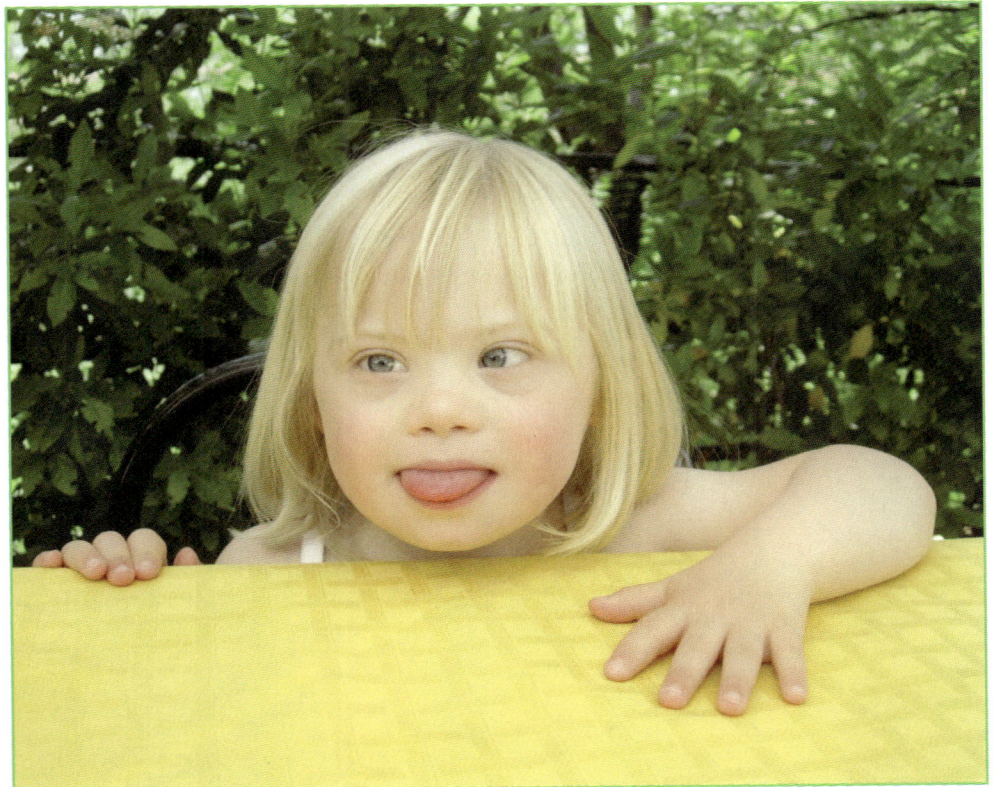

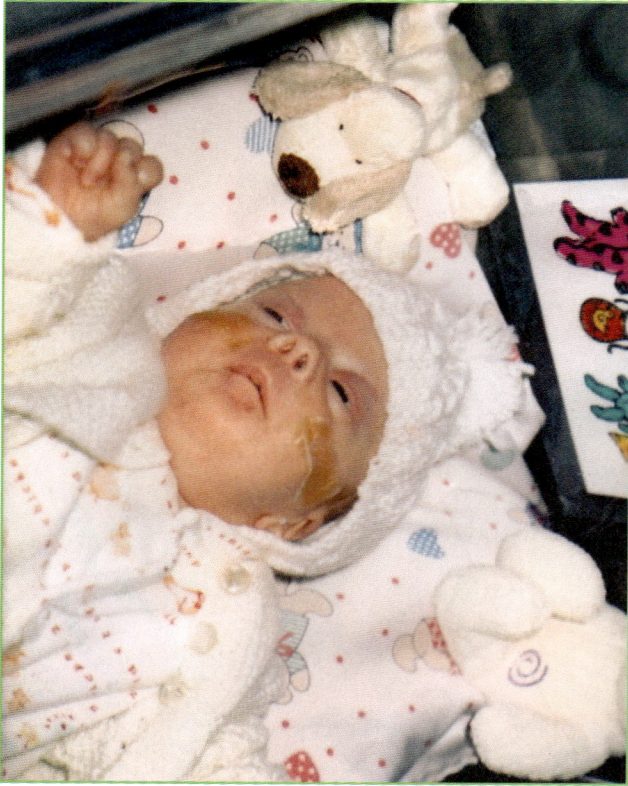

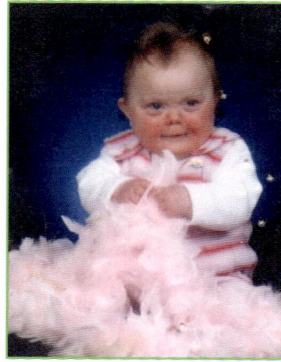

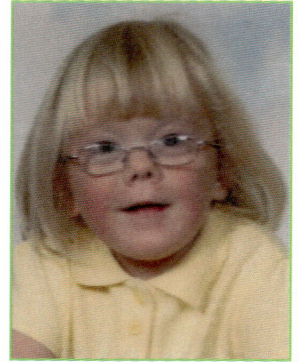

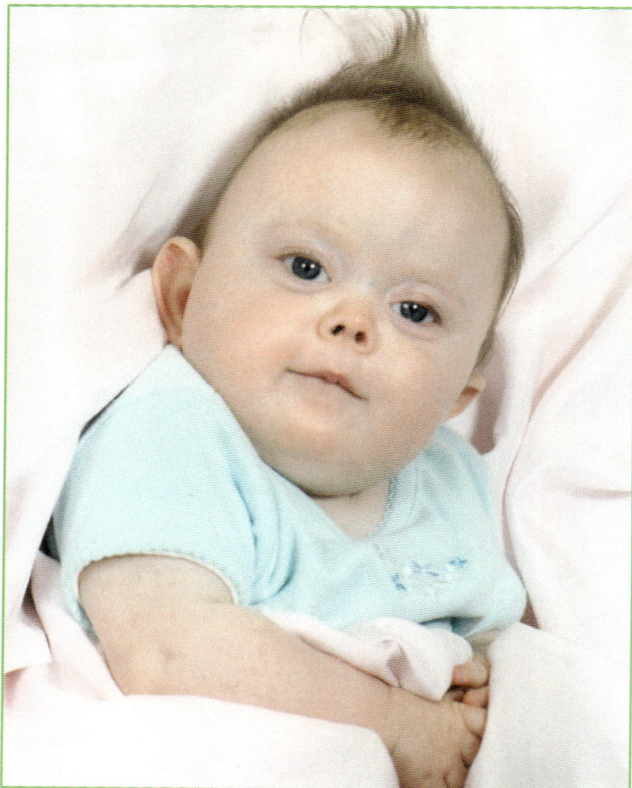

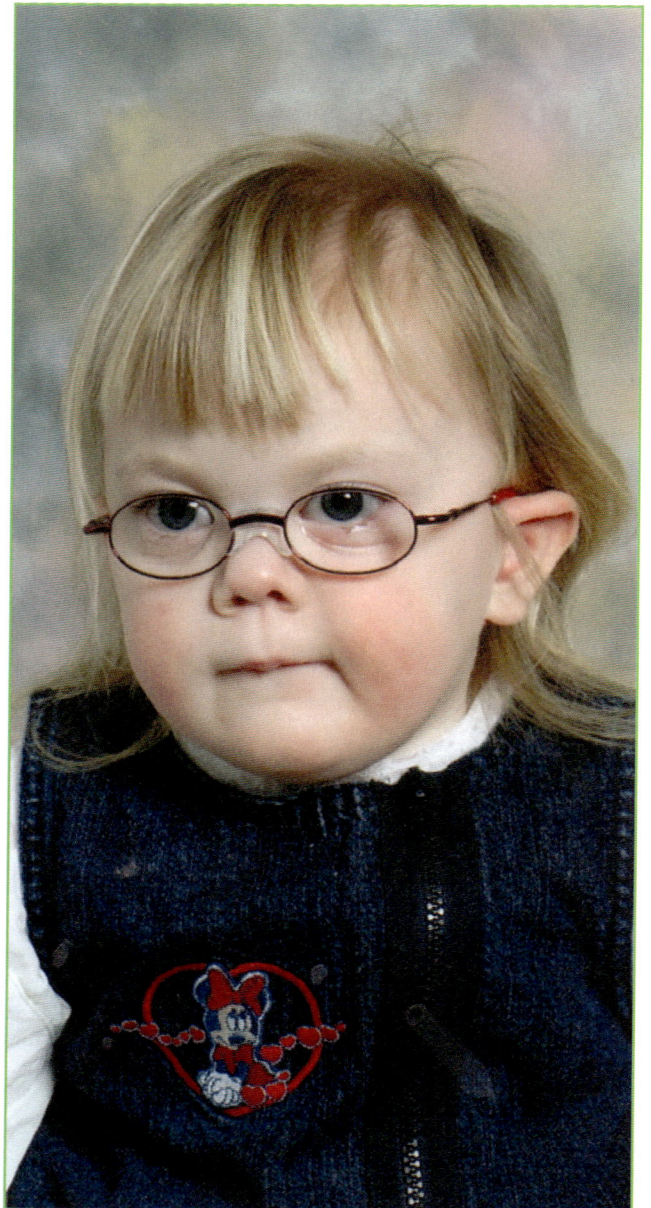

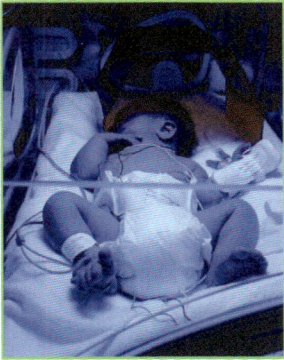

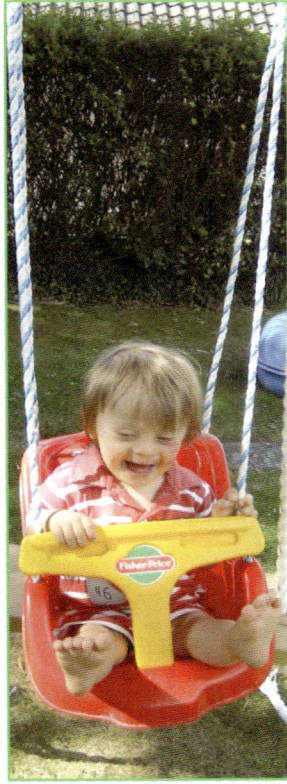

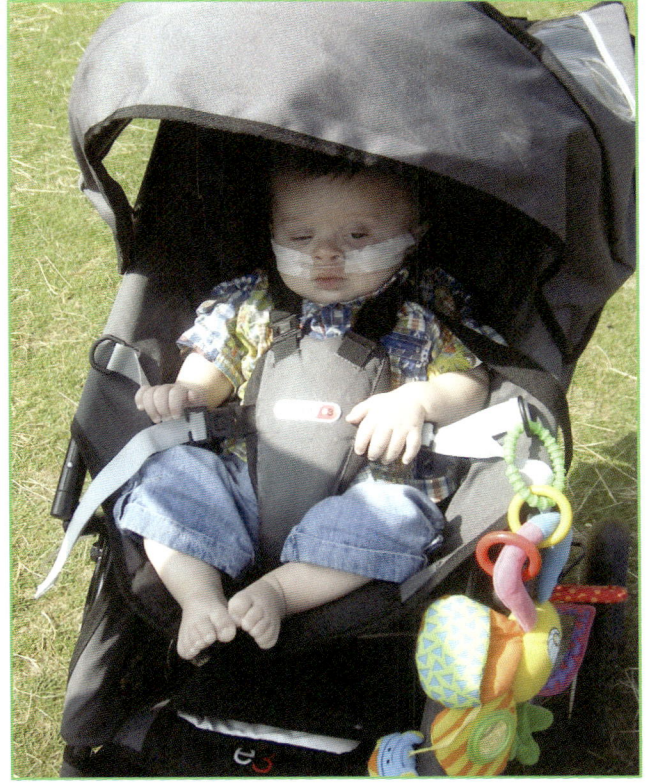

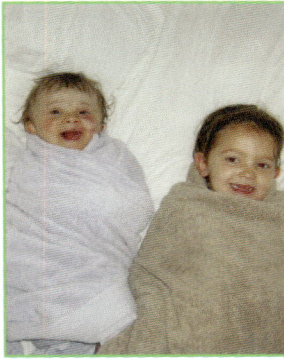

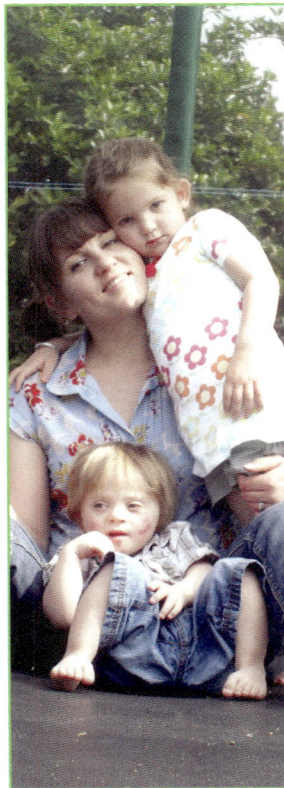

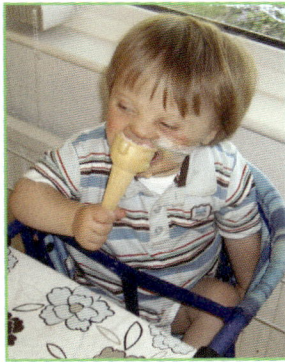

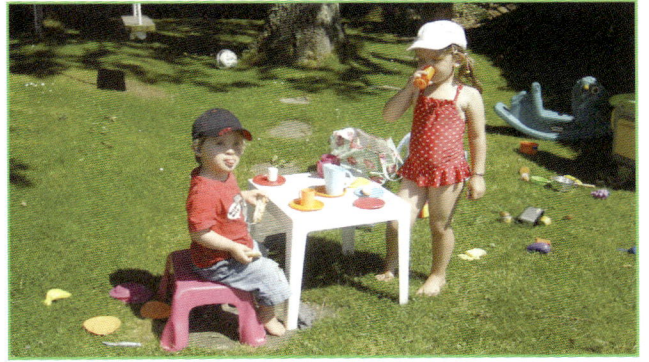

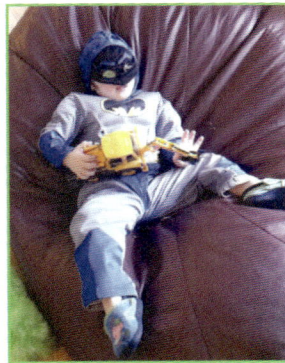

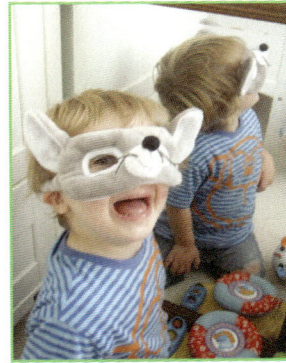

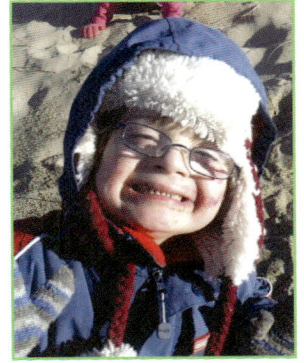

William

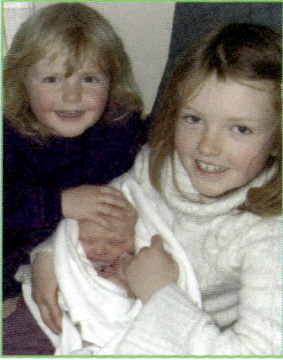
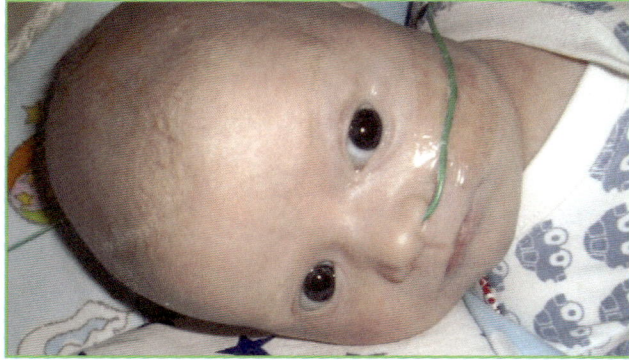
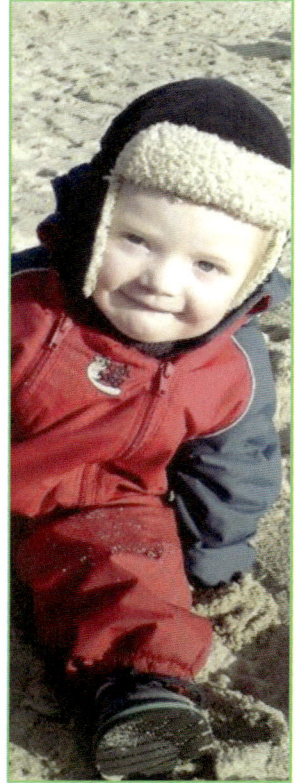
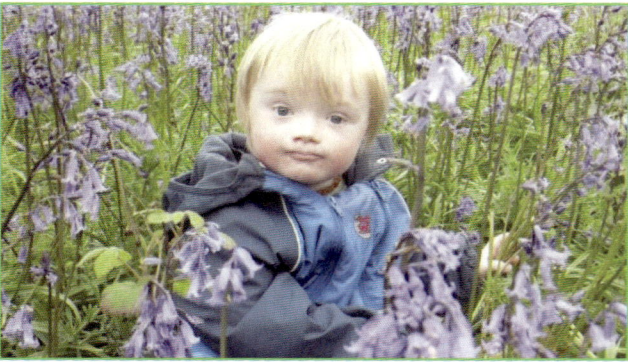
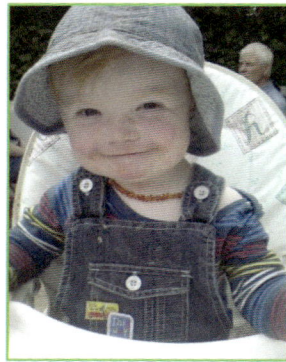
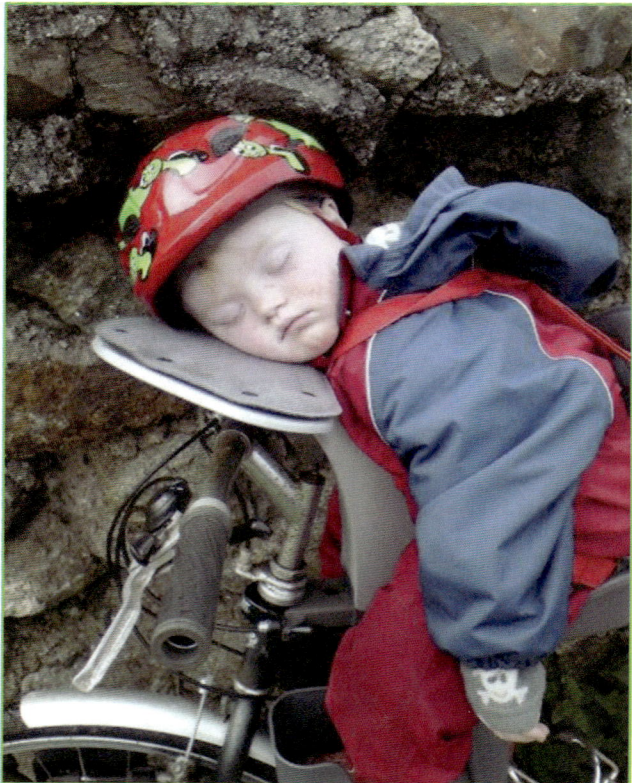
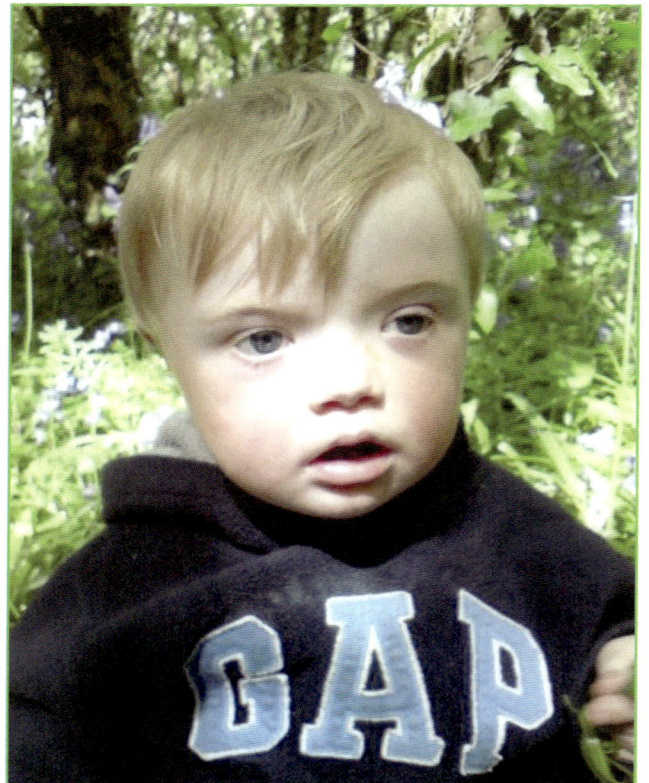

The close bond of a personal friendship inspired Simon and Anna Burt to invite the Cornwall Down's Syndrome Support Group into their Truro photography studio. The project aimed for diagnosis to feature as a secondary aspect and as a result they were able to create a portrait collection depicting the fun and colourful character of each individual.

"It's not what you look at that matters, but what you see"

David Henry Thoreau

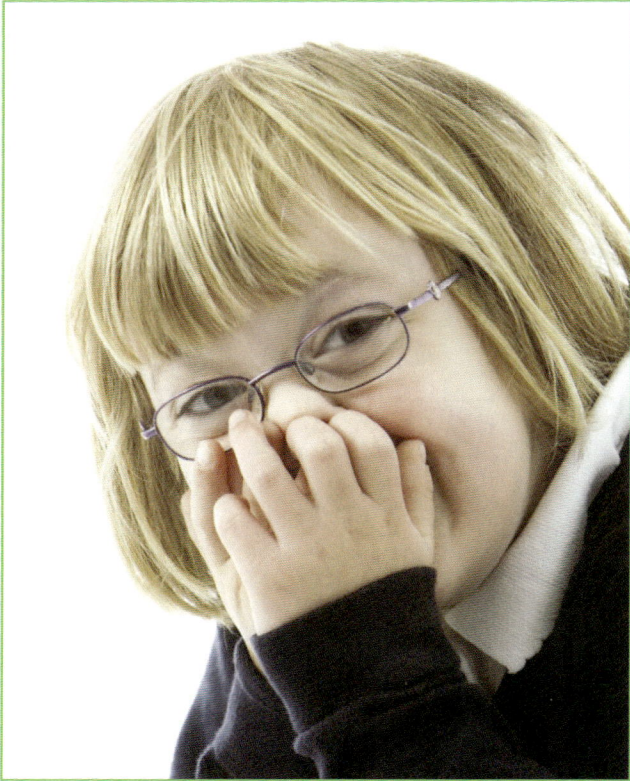

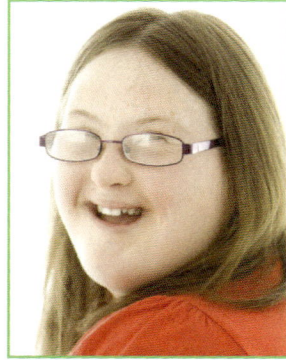

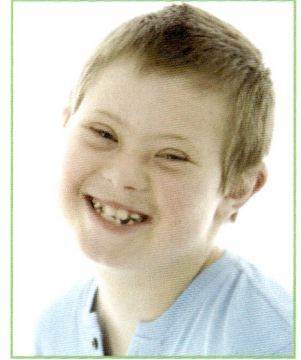

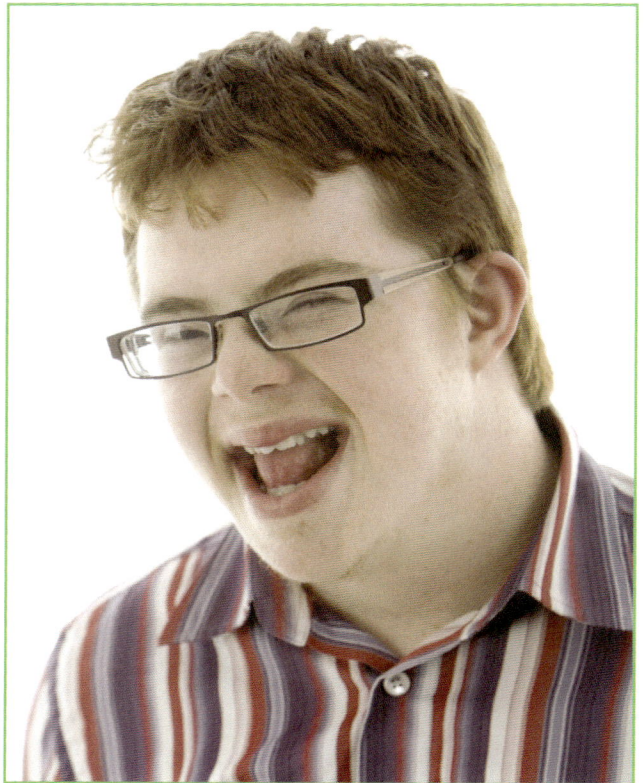

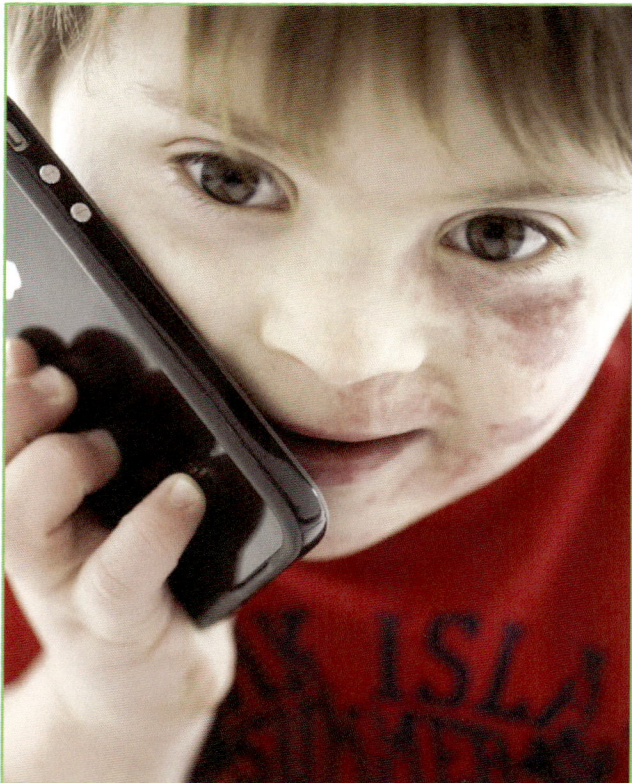

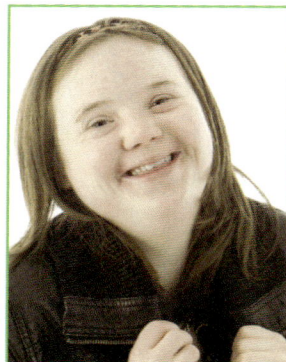

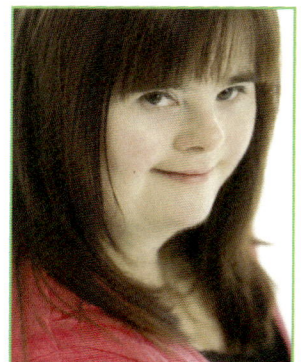

Photographs by Simon Burt www.simonburtphotography.co.uk

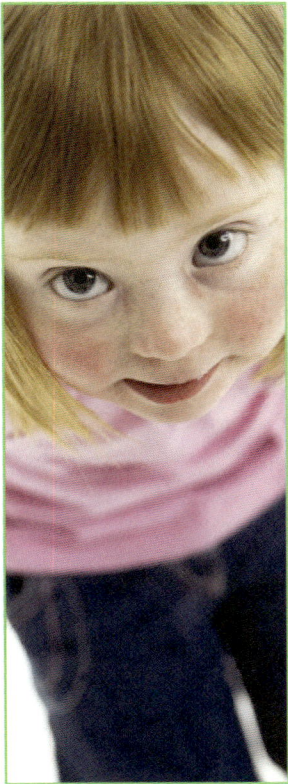

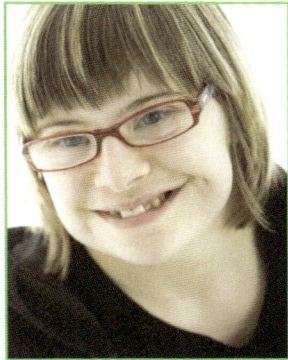

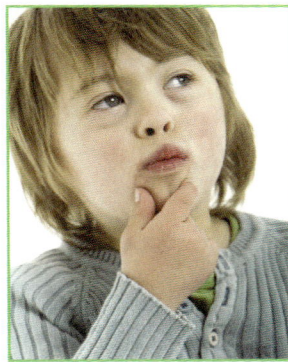

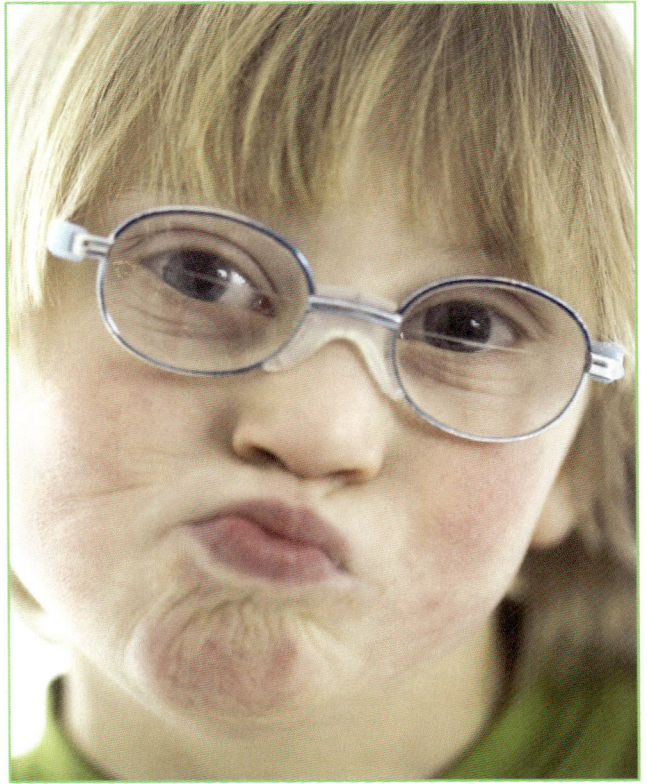

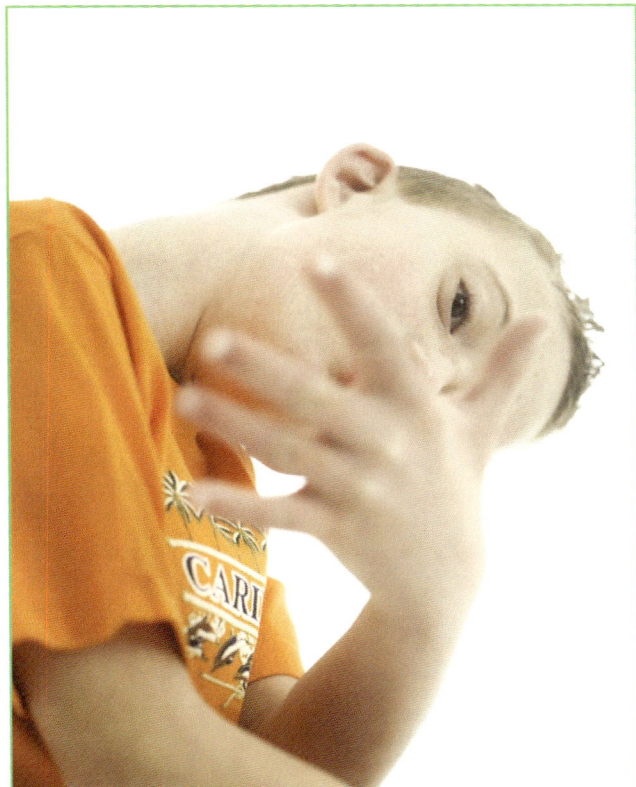

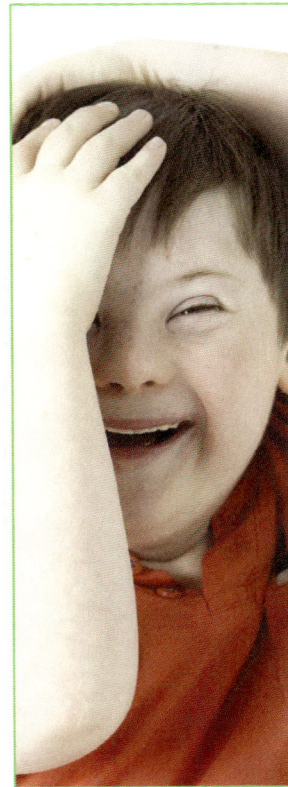

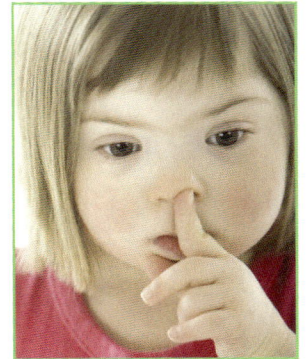

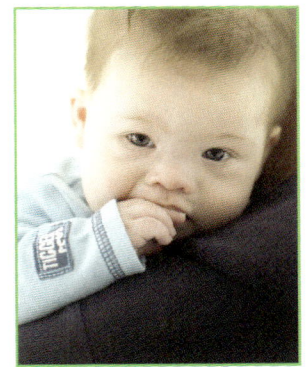

Lightning Source UK Ltd.
Milton Keynes UK
UKIC02n0829020615
252716UK00006B/7

9 780956 936738